Understanding the

MENOPAUSE

D1347848

Published by Family Doctor Publicati
in association with the British Medic

Family Doctor Publications, PO Box 4664, Poole, Dorset BH15 1NN

Medical Editor: Dr Tony Smith
Cover Artist: Dave Eastbury
Medical Artist: Peter Cox Associates
Design: Peter Powell Origination & Print Limited
Printing: Nuffield Press, Abingdon, Oxon, using acid-free paper

ISBN: 1 903474 11 6

Contents

The menopause: what happens to your body?

The word 'menopause' strictly means a woman's last menstrual period, which typically occurs around the age of 51, and defines the end of the fertile phase of a woman's life. The 'change of life' or 'climacteric' is the time when your body is adjusting before, during and after the menopause. There are hormonal changes and symptoms in the years leading up to, and beyond, your final menstrual period. It has been estimated that, by the age of 54 years, most women (80 per cent) have had their last menstrual period – they are then termed postmenopausal.

Some women experience a natural menopause before the age of 40. This is considered premature. Menopause can be induced prematurely by radiotherapy or chemotherapy used to treat some cancers, or following surgery to remove the ovaries. In such women, hot flushes and sweats can be particularly severe.

Many women adjust to the changes without problems and some revel in their new-found freedom – free from the monthly 'curse' of periods, particularly if periods were painful or heavy, and free from the fear of unwanted pregnancy. However, not all women find the change of life easy and, although some may benefit from self-help treatments, others need medical support.

HORMONAL CHANGES

From puberty to the menopause, women's bodies follow hormonal cycles – the monthly periods. Each month the levels of the female hormone, oestrogen, rise over the early part of the cycle, stimulating the growth of an egg, which is released from one of the two ovaries at mid-cycle. Following ovulation, another female hormone, progesterone, stimulates the lining of the uterus to thicken, ready for a possible pregnancy. If the egg is not fertilised by sperm, it dies and the egg and uterus lining are shed as a period.

In the years leading up to the menopause, the ovaries become less efficient, resulting in irregular and often heavy periods. Eventually, they stop functioning, no further eggs are released and periods stop. At the same time, the monthly hormonal cycle becomes more erratic. Blood levels of oestrogen fluctuate – low levels give rise to hot flushes, night sweats and many other symptoms.

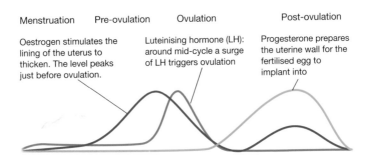

Menstruation   Pre-ovulation   Ovulation   Post-ovulation

Oestrogen stimulates the lining of the uterus to thicken. The level peaks just before ovulation.

Luteinising hormone (LH): around mid-cycle a surge of LH triggers ovulation

Progesterone prepares the uterine wall for the fertilised egg to implant into

The principal changes in hormones during the menstrual cycle

Menstrual bleeding

Unfertilised egg from last menstrual cycle leaves uterus

Endometrium (lining of the uterus) doubles in thickness, in response to hormones

0 2 4 6 8 10 11 12 14 16 18 20 22 24 26 28

Changes in the lining of the uterus during the menstrual cycle

Changes during the menstrual cycle.

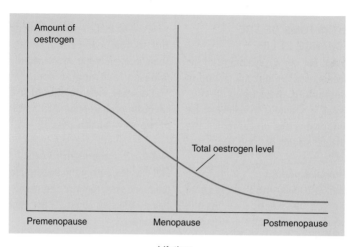

Lifetime

Oestrogen levels gradually decline towards the menopause. After the menopause the ovaries cease functioning, oestrogen levels fall and periods stop.

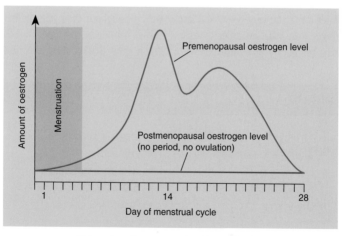

Pre- and postmenopausal oestrogen levels.

Until the menopause, women produce oestrogen in varying amounts over a 28-day cycle. However, after the menopause, oestrogen production falls to a low level and this increases the risk of bone fractures, strokes and heart disease.

Symptoms of the 'change in life'

Most, but not all, symptoms of the menopause are directly related to fluctuating oestrogen levels. Possible solutions to relieve these symptoms are discussed in the chapter starting on page 10.

Irregular periods

This is usually the first sign that signals the menopause. As the ovaries become erratic in their production of oestrogen and progesterone, so your menstrual cycle becomes irregular. At first your cycle typically shortens from its usual 28 days to between 21 and 25 days. Later on, it lengthens, with occasional skipped periods. Your period itself can change – sometimes it may be very heavy and last longer than usual, at other times it may be scanty and short. Fewer cycles result in the release of an egg and so you become less fertile. Sometimes an egg is spontaneously released following an apparent menopause, so you should use adequate contraception until a year or two after your final period.

Hot flushes and night sweats

Hot flushes and night sweats are hallmark symptoms of the menopause, affecting about 75 per cent of women.

Flushes often start around the age of 47 or 48 and usually continue for three or four years. In the early stages of the menopause they may occur only in the week before menstruation, when oestrogen levels are naturally low. Eventually, oestrogen levels fluctuate sufficiently throughout the cycle so that flushes happen at any time. Flushes reach their peak during the first

SYMPTOMS OF THE MENOPAUSE

- Anxiety
- Changes to skin and hair
- Depression
- Disrupted sleep
- Dry vagina
- Fatigue
- Headaches
- Hot flushes and night sweats
- Irregular periods
- Irritability
- Joint and muscle pain
- Loss of interest in sex
- Painful intercourse
- Palpitations
- Poor concentration
- Poor memory
- Urinary problems

couple of years after the last menstrual period, and then ease over time. In some women flushes start earlier; for some it happens in their late 30s or early 40s. Flushes can continue for 5 or 10 years; 25 per cent of women will have occasional flushes for more than 5 years. A Swedish study found that about 9 per cent of 72-year-old women have hot flushes.

Many women can sense when a flush is about to start, often noticing a feeling of increasing pressure in the head and a faster pulse. Within a few minutes, the flush rapidly spreads across the shoulders and chest, rising up the neck and head. This often causes great discomfort and embarrassment. Flushes usually last a matter of seconds but can persist for 15 minutes or so, recurring several times during the day. You might also notice sweating or palpitations and feel weak or faint. Night sweats can be particularly severe, disrupting sleep – some women have to change their nightclothes and even their sheets because they wake drenched in sweat.

Disrupted sleep

Symptoms such as night sweats are not the only reason for disrupted sleep. Such symptoms can also be a symptom of underlying anxiety or depression. Anxiety usually causes difficulty getting to sleep – you feel extremely tired but your mind keeps ticking over the events of the day or you worry about the future. Depression is more often associated with early morning waking – you get to sleep without too much trouble but wake in the early hours tossing and turning until it is time to get up.

As the hormonal changes of the menopause can aggravate underlying anxiety and depression, specific medical treatment for these conditions may be necessary. So, if sleepless nights continue, particularly if you have successfully controlled other symptoms of the 'change', you should seek help from your doctor.

Headaches

Fluctuating hormone levels can trigger migraine and other headaches in susceptible women. During the 'change' women notice an increasing link between headaches and their monthly periods. Premenstrual symptoms, that is, occurring a week or two before a period, become more prominent at this time of life and both migraine and non-migraine headaches can worsen during the premenstrual week. Headaches usually improve when hormonal fluctuations settle after the menopause. If the headaches are troublesome, your doctor or a specialist headache clinic can advise on specific treatment.

Joint and muscle pains

Aching wrists, knees and ankles, and lower back pain are common and may often be confused with arthritis.

Painful intercourse

Oestrogen stimulates the production of mucus, which keeps the vagina and other sexual parts moist. After the menopause, lack of oestrogen means that less lubricating mucus is produced. The vagina becomes shorter, less elastic and dryer. As well as intercourse becoming more painful, these changes can result in itching and irritation. However, sexual excitement stimulates the production of lubricating fluids, so prolonged foreplay can help prevent painful intercourse.

Loss of libido

Sexual desire frequently lessens with the menopause and it often takes longer to become aroused. Sexual desire is also affected by general well-being, emotional upsets and painful intercourse.

Urinary symptoms

A sudden need to urinate (urge incontinence), even when you have just been to the toilet, is a common problem after the menopause; lack of oestrogen causes the tissues around the neck of the bladder to thin. Also the muscles that support the uterus and prevent the bladder from leaking become weaker.

Coughing and running typically provoke an embarrassing leak of urine (stress incontinence), which affects between 10 and 20 per cent of women over 60 and up to 40 per cent of women in their 80s. Stress incontinence also commonly affects women in their late 40s and throughout their 50s

Recurring urine infections are also more common as the skin around the bladder becomes thinner and drier. Oestrogen deficiency changes the acidity of the vaginal secretions, resulting in fewer of the protective bacteria being present that help to fight off infection before the menopause. A common sign of possible infection is burning or stinging when urinating.

Dry skin and hair

Oestrogen keeps your skin moist and stimulates hair growth – hence the 'bloom' of pregnancy when oestrogen levels are very high. Without oestrogen your skin becomes dry, losing its suppleness so that wrinkles become more prominent. Hair growth slows but the rate of hair loss stays the same so your hair becomes thinner and less manageable.

Dry eyes

As well as skin becoming drier after the menopause, many women notice that their eyes become persistently dry and itchy as fewer tears are produced.

Weight gain

Women may put on weight because of reduced physical activity – perhaps just as a result of lifestyle changes but maybe because of joint problems. As we age our bodies burn up energy more slowly than when we were younger, which can also lead to weight gain if we don't either eat less or exercise more. Hormonal changes also play a role, because oestrogen is responsible for maintaining the female shape; after the menopause weight tends to settle more around the waist than the hips.

Emotional symptoms

Poor sleep has a knock-on effect resulting in daytime tiredness, lethargy, difficulty concentrating and depression. These symptoms are often very distressing and make it even harder to cope with daily demands. Finding ways to improve sleep, either by controlling the flushes or by treating depression, can help restore the balance.

Non-hormonal symptoms

Depression and sexual problems around the menopause are not just the result of falling levels of oestrogen. The menopause marks a time in a woman's life that can be difficult for many reasons – it may coincide with children leaving home, impending retirement, marital difficulties, ill or dying parents.

These changes take their own toll and may need professional support. Some women may benefit from professional support which is available through GPs

DIAGNOSING THE 'CHANGE'

The symptoms of the 'change' are usually sufficient evidence to make the diagnosis, particularly for women in their late 40s or early 50s. If there is any uncertainty about the diagnosis, for example if a woman experiences an unusually early menopause, the diagnosis can be confirmed by a simple blood test to check the hormone levels. Unless a woman's periods have stopped completely, the blood tests are usually taken within the first week of the menstrual cycle, the first day of the cycle being the first day of bleeding. These tests check the levels of follicle-stimulating homone (FSH) and luteinising hormone (LH), which are higher than usual if a woman is perimenopausal (close to the menopause). Sometimes a second test is taken about a week before the expected start of menstruation to measure the levels of progesterone. The presence of this hormone confirms that the woman has ovulated that cycle. As these blood tests give a result only for that particular menstrual cycle, and normal hormone surges can occasionally confuse the results, the results

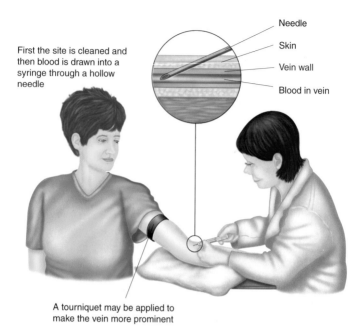

First the site is cleaned and then blood is drawn into a syringe through a hollow needle

Needle

Skin

Vein wall

Blood in vein

A tourniquet may be applied to make the vein more prominent

The menopause can be confirmed by a simple blood test to check the hormone levels.

must be viewed in the context of all the symptoms – a single normal result does not exclude the menopause.

POSTMENOPAUSAL RISKS

The menopause has taken on much greater importance over recent years, particularly in western society, because, with a life expectancy of over 80 years (and rising), many women can expect to be postmenopausal for over one-third of their lives.

Although the symptoms of the climacteric are not life threatening, the long-term effects of oestrogen deficiency can be. The major diseases of old age are heart disease, strokes, breast and bowel cancer, osteoporosis and fractures, and dementia. All of these are affected by oestrogen so women with a premature menopause are at particular risk. Although these conditions do not always result in death, they may lead to a significant reduction in quality of life, for both the individuals affected and their relatives.

KEY POINTS

✓ There are many symptoms of the 'change' and they vary from mild to severe

✓ Typical symptoms are irregular periods, hot flushes and night sweats

✓ Symptoms can also include mood changes, difficulty sleeping and depression

✓ Diagnosis of the menopause is usually based on the symptoms

✓ Most symptoms settle within a few years of periods stopping

✓ Women now live longer and the long-term effects of oestrogen deficiency are increasingly apparent; the risk of fractures, strokes and heart disease increases with each year after the menopause

Helping yourself to feel better

MENOPAUSAL SYMPTOMS

Simple measures are worth trying before complementary or prescription therapies are considered, particularly if the symptoms are relatively mild.

Flushes and sweats

Keep cool – hot flushes can be triggered by a rise in temperature, eating hot spicy foods, or hot drinks such as tea or coffee. Anecdotally, women report that using a fan and drinking cold drinks can help. Wear natural fibres that allow air to circulate around the skin and layer thinner clothes rather than wearing one thick sweater. Use cotton sheets or duvet covers and sleep in a cool room with adequate ventilation.

- **Exercise:** Physically active women experience fewer and less severe flushes than sedentary women.

- **Lose weight:** A high body mass predisposes to more frequent and severe flushes.

- **Stop smoking:** The more a women smokes, the more flushes she is likely to have.

- **Relax:** Slow, controlled breathing can reduce the severity of a flush when performed as soon as a flush begins.

Disrupted sleep

The above strategies of exercise, weight loss and relaxation similarly apply to improving sleep. Avoid stimulating food and drink near bedtime, particularly alcohol – try a warm milky drink instead. Have a warm bath and read a book or watch TV until you feel sleepy, but beware of thrillers and other stimulating programmes! Keep the room cool with circulating fresh air. If you wake in the night and cannot go back to sleep, get up, make a drink and read for a while. If you feel tired during the day, take a 20-minute nap – longer than this will make it harder to sleep at night.

Irregular periods

As periods become more irregular, they often also become heavier and more painful. Mild period problems can be helped by gentle exercise or heat but heavy, painful periods often require specific treatment. If simple painkillers don't help, visit the doctor for advice. As heavy periods can lead to anaemia, boost iron intake with iron-rich foods such as meat and spinach, or with iron supplements.

Headaches

Most headaches result from some obvious underlying cause such as missed meals, lack of sleep or muscular pain. Migraine headaches can arise from similar triggers so help reduce frequent attacks by eating regularly and getting enough sleep. Simple painkillers or over-the-counter migraine treatments help to control symptoms but follow the instructions and do not take them for more than a couple of days a week; more frequent use can exacerbate the problem as rebound symptoms occur. Also, frequent use of painkillers can suppress the body's own natural painkillers, the endorphins, increasing pain. If headaches do not respond to simple measures, see a doctor who can advise on treatment, including drugs to treat and to prevent attacks. For more information on headaches see the Family Doctor book *Understanding Migraine and Other Headaches.*

Joint and muscle pains

Deep-heat creams and gels or a heat-pad can give some relief but painkillers, such as paracetamol, or anti-inflammatory drugs, such as aspirin or ibuprofen, may be necessary if your symptoms are severe. If these are not effective, seek the advice of a general practitioner. Try gentle, non-weight-bearing exercise such as cycling or swimming. Losing weight can reduce the load on your joints. Fish oil supplements and glucosamine may help.

Vaginal dryness

If vaginal dryness is the only problem, lubricating gels may help. They can be bought from a pharmacy. Never use petroleum jelly, or other oil-based products, because these prevent air reaching the skin and increase the risk of infections. Smear the product liberally over the vulval area, particularly round the opening of the vagina. Replens and Senselle are artificial lubricants that are used two or three times a week. They coat the inside of the vagina with a non-hormonal moisturiser, which lasts for a day or two, so they do not have to be used immediately before intercourse. In contrast, KY jelly needs to be used just before intercourse.

Loss of libido
Sex drive naturally lessens over the years and it takes longer to get aroused. Whereas younger women may become sufficiently aroused for penetrative sex in as short a time as a few seconds, menopausal women may take five minutes or more. Taking time during sex, with lots of foreplay, enables the Bartholin's glands to produce the maximum amount of lubrication before penetration.

Urinary symptoms
Simply crossing the legs when you feel a cough or sneeze starting can help prevent leakage. Eat plenty of fresh fruit, vegetables and fibre to avoid constipation, which can cause pressure on the bladder and urethra. Also try to lose weight, because being overweight puts

stress on the pelvic floor muscles. These muscles provide support to the bladder, rectum and uterus. They are weakened by childbirth and are further weakened by oestrogen deficiency after the menopause. Strengthening the muscles can help reduce leakage.

The most common technique is pelvic floor exercises, sometimes known as Kegel exercises after their inventor Dr Arnold Kegel. You may have to do them for a few months before you notice any improvement. You can do them at any time – while driving the car, doing the housework, talking on the phone. Sit with your knees slightly apart and imagine that you are trying to stop yourself passing wind from the back passage; to do this you must tighten the muscles round your back passage. Squeeze and lift those muscles as if you really do have wind: you should be able to feel the muscles move and the skin round the back passage tightening. Your legs and buttocks should not move at all. Then imagine that you are sitting on the toilet urinating. Imagine yourself trying to stop the stream of urine. Hold the muscles tight for at least five seconds if you can, then relax. Repeat at least five times. Now pull the muscles up quickly and tightly. Repeat at least five times. Do these exercises – five slow and five fast – at least ten times every day.

Weak pelvic floor muscles

Low bladder neck

Before exercise

Raised bladder neck

Contracting pelvic floor muscles

After exercise

Pelvic floor exercises re-educate and strengthen the muscles in the pelvic floor, and so increase support for the bladder and urethra.

Small weighted plastic cones inserted into the vagina, which can be bought from the chemist, can help exercise the correct muscles, because the pelvic floor muscles have to be tensed to prevent the cones falling out.

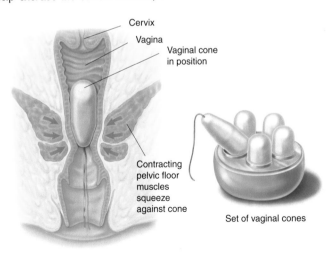

Cervix

Vagina

Vaginal cone in position

Contracting pelvic floor muscles squeeze against cone

Set of vaginal cones

Weighted vaginal cones can be used to strengthen the pelvic floor muscles.

If you find these exercises difficult or ineffective, your doctor can give advice or may refer you to a specialist continence adviser.

Do not restrict the amount of fluids you drink as this can worsen the problem by increasing your susceptibility to cystitis because harmful bacteria are less likely to be urinated away. But do cut out coffee, strong tea and other caffeine-rich drinks, such as fizzy cola, that stimulate the bladder muscle.

Cystitis may respond to treatments from the chemist containing sodium citrate, which makes the urine less acidic. Alternatively, drink cranberry juice or water with a teaspoon of bicarbonate of soda added which also makes the urine less acidic. If your symptoms do not ease within a day or so, see your doctor as you may have an infection and need antibiotics.

Dry skin and hair
Keep to a simple haircut that is easy to manage and use conditioner to stop your hair becoming too dry. If you are out in the sun, use an effective sun cream and wear a hat.

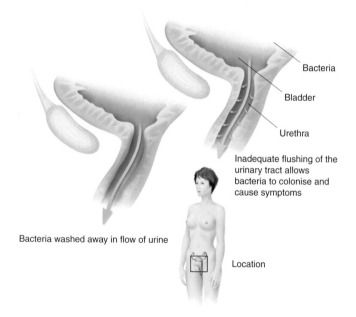

Bacteria

Bladder

Urethra

Inadequate flushing of the urinary tract allows bacteria to colonise and cause symptoms

Bacteria washed away in flow of urine

Location

Infections do not usually take hold in the urinary tract because bacteria are constantly flushed away by the flow of urine; the immune system is generally able to cope with the few bacteria that do creep in.

If you swim regularly, wear a swimming hat and apply plenty of moisturiser after showering, as chlorine is very drying to both skin and hair.

Dry eyes
Women frequently experience problems with dry eyes as they enter the menopause. Many find relief simply from using artificial tears that can be bought from a pharmacy. There are a variety of different chemicals used, including hypromellose, hydroxyethylcellulose, liquid paraffin or saline solution. Preservative-free tears are the most soothing. Avoid products that whiten the eyes – they do not have adequate lubricating qualities and often make the problem worse. Simple lifestyle changes can significantly improve irritation from dry eyes; for example, drinking eight to ten glasses of water spaced over the course of each day keeps the body hydrated. Make a conscious effort to blink frequently – especially when reading, working at the computer or watching television. Avoid rubbing the eyes as it only worsens the irritation.

If simple remedies are not effective, see a doctor – certain medications, thyroid conditions, vitamin A deficiency and diseases such as Parkinson's disease and Sjögren's syndrome, a condition where the immune system attacks the glands that produce tears and saliva, can also cause dryness.

Weight gain
Increasing evidence suggests that postmenopausal weight gain is nature's way of producing more oestrogen. After the menopause a certain amount of oestrogen is formed in fat, so the fatter you are, the more oestrogen you produce. This may explain why, in general, fat women have stronger bones than thin women. Obviously, a balance is necessary because obesity is linked to heart disease. The simple message is that, in most cases, keeping fit and eating a healthy balanced diet allow weight to settle at its natural level.

Emotional symptoms
Most of us have felt low at some time in our lives. Usually it is the result of a particular event, and these feelings eventually ease with time. Hormonal changes can make it harder to cope. Finding ways to relax and unwind, eating healthily and taking adequate exercise will all improve mood. Limit consumption of alcohol because it can aggravate depression. Seek medical help early – a supportive doctor may be all that is needed, but counselling or drug therapy may be necessary.

PREVENTING HEART DISEASE AND OSTEOPOROSIS

What is heart disease?

The heart is essentially a muscle that pumps blood around the body. Blood vessels, or arteries, supply blood to the heart muscle. When blood flow through the arteries becomes obstructed, the heart muscle can die – this is when a heart attack occurs. The most common way such obstructions develop is through a condition called atherosclerosis, a largely preventable disease. Blood vessels to the brain can also be affected by atherosclerosis, which can result in strokes.

Lifestyle changes to prevent heart disease

Many of the risk factors for heart disease can be reduced by simple lifestyle changes: losing weight, stopping smoking, modifying diet and taking more exercise.

What is osteoporosis?

Osteoporosis is a disease in which bones become fragile and more likely to break. Unfortunately there are no symptoms of osteoporosis until a bone breaks. These broken bones, known as fractures, typically affect the hip, spine, and wrist.

A hip fracture can cause prolonged or permanent disability or even death. Spinal or vertebral fractures also have serious consequences, including loss of height, severe back pain and deformity.

Lifestyle changes to prevent osteoporosis

Adequate exercise and a healthy calcium-rich diet keep bones strong. Effective prevention of osteoporosis starts early, however, preferably in childhood – there is plenty that can be done to protect children. They need exercise and a good diet including calcium-rich foods, and should be warned about the hazards of smoking. Peak adult bone mass is reached around the age of 35. The peak bone mass for men is 25 to 30 per cent greater than for women, placing women at greater risk of osteoporosis. Bone loss starts shortly after the peak, starting earlier in women than in men, and is accelerated by the menopause.

Exercise for a healthy heart and strong bones

The value of exercise cannot be overemphasised. Studies show that being physically fit lowers heart disease risk even in people who have other health problems such as high blood pressure and high cholesterol. To minimise risk, however, you should be physically fit and avoid the other major modifiable risk factors: cigarette smoke, high blood pressure and high blood cholesterol.

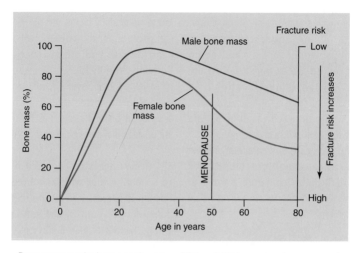

Bone mass peaks between the ages of 25 and 40 in men and women and then starts to fall. In women, accelerated loss of bone mass occurs around the time of the menopause.

It is never too late to start exercising – one study showed that an 80 year old gains the same percentage improvement in muscle strength as a 25 year old. If you are inactive, doing anything is better than nothing! Studies show that people who have a low fitness level are much more likely to die earlier than people who have achieved even a moderate level of fitness. It is not just your heart and bones that benefit from regular exercise; muscle strength and power also improve, making falls less likely and, if you do trip, you have more strength to grab on to something. If you take drugs such as tranquillisers, hypnotics or alcohol, reassess your need for them as they may

affect your judgement, making you more likely to trip or stumble.

Weight-bearing exercise strengthens bone and can also help to prevent fractures. The easiest and most convenient exercise is walking – which strengths your heart and bones. Start gently and gradually increase the distance. Swimming is not weight bearing because the body is supported by the water, but it is excellent if you have joint problems and is also good for the heart.

Although the ideal recommendation for exercise is 20 to 30 minutes of brisk activity, three times a week, this need not be as daunting as it sounds. When done for as little as 30 minutes a day, activities such as climbing stairs, gardening, moderate-to-heavy housework, dancing and home exercise are all beneficial. Again, doing anything is better than nothing.

Middle-aged or older people who are inactive and at high risk for heart disease or who already have a medical condition should seek medical advice before starting or significantly increasing their physical activity.

Exercise as a daily routine

The main reason why people fail to take exercise is simply a lack of time to incorporate exercise into their daily routine. Why not walk or cycle to the shops instead of taking the bus or car; if it is too far, get off the bus one stop earlier, or park your car further away. If you feel up to more formal exercise, such as jogging, go ahead but be careful not to overdo it in the early stages.

Always warm up and cool down gradually to prevent injury to muscles. Avoid vigorous exercise if you are unwell because it can put an undue strain on your heart. Remember, an exercise programme should be maintained for life, not just for a few weeks a year.

Watch your diet

• **Natural oestrogens:** Some studies suggest that natural oestrogens found in many plant foods, particularly beans and pulses, can protect against osteoporosis, heart disease and breast cancer. Certainly, the incidence of these diseases is much lower in countries such as Japan where oestrogen-rich soya bean products, such as tofu, are an essential part of the diet.

• **Calcium:** Bones contain calcium, so a healthy diet with adequate calcium is necessary to ensure that bones develop properly and remain strong. Periods of growth obviously increase the relative demands for calcium, so teenagers and pregnant women need greater amounts. The recommended daily amount for adults is 700 milligrams (mg). Dairy foods such as milk, cheese and yoghurt are the best sources of calcium, which is readily absorbed into the bloodstream. Unfortunately, the current fashion for dieting has meant that many women cut out dairy products because they also contain high levels of fat. The answer is to continue eating dairy products but switch to low-fat alternatives – skimmed milk actually contains slightly more calcium than whole milk. Tinned bony fish such as sardines or salmon are excellent because the softened bones are rich in calcium.

• **Vitamin D:** This vitamin helps the absorption of calcium. Dietary intake of vitamin D has declined over the

DIETARY SOURCES OF CALCIUM

Dairy products (average portion)	Calcium content (milligrams or mg)	Non-dairy products (average portion)	Calcium content (mg)
Skimmed milk: 190 millilitres or ml (third of a pint)	235	Tofu (steamed): 100 g	510
Semi-skimmed milk: 190 ml (third of a pint)	231	Sardines in oil (drained): 60 g	220
Whole milk: 190 ml (third of a pint)	224	Dried figs: 30 g	75
Yoghurt: 140 g (5 oz)	240	Baked beans: 120 g (4 oz)	50
Edam cheese: 30 g (1 oz)	216	1 orange	47
Cheddar cheese: 30 g (1 oz)	207	1 slice of white bread	28
Cottage cheese: 30 g (1 oz)	82	1 slice of brown bread	7

years and may be linked to increasing fracture rates. Fatty fish, such as halibut, mackerel and salmon, are rich sources of vitamin D; studies suggest that two meals of fatty fish a week can reduce the fracture risk by up to 20 per cent.

• **Supplementing your diet:** Calcium supplements are a useful addition to a poor diet, particularly in early life when bones are developing. If you have been diagnosed with osteoporosis you will need to supplement your diet to ensure that you get around 1,000–1,200 mg of calcium daily. Vitamin D is also available as supplements of 400–800 international units or IU (10–20 micrograms) daily. It is often combined with calcium. Be careful not to overdo it – taking more than 2,000 mg of calcium can increase your risk of kidney stones and may interfere with your absorption of other minerals such as iron.

Cut down on alcohol

Although moderate drinking is thought to be beneficial to health, heavy drinking increases your risk of osteoporosis and heart disease in addition to its effects on general health. The density of the hip bone is reduced by up to 12 per cent in women in their late 40s who regularly drink more than two units of alcohol a day, so try to drink no more than this. One unit is equivalent to a small glass of wine, a single measure of spirits or half a pint of beer.

Control your weight

Middle-aged spread can help maintain bone density, because hormones produced by the adrenal gland and the postmenopausal ovaries are converted to oestrogen in fat cells. However, it is important to keep a healthy weight because being overweight is associated with increased risk of heart disease and strokes.

The body mass index (BMI) is a useful index of healthy weight and is easily calculated if you know your

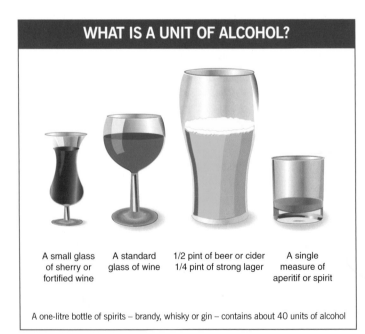

WHAT IS A UNIT OF ALCOHOL?

A small glass of sherry or fortified wine

A standard glass of wine

1/2 pint of beer or cider 1/4 pint of strong lager

A single measure of aperitif or spirit

A one-litre bottle of spirits – brandy, whisky or gin – contains about 40 units of alcohol

WHAT SHOULD YOU WEIGH?

- The body mass index (BMI) is a useful measure of healthy weight
- Find out your height in metres and weight in kilograms
- Calculate your BMI like this:

$$BMI = \frac{\text{Your weight (kg)}}{[\text{Your height (metres) x your height (metres)}]}$$

$$e.g.\ 24.8 = \frac{70}{[1.68 \times 1.68]}$$

- You are recommended to try to maintain a BMI in the range 20–25
- The chart below is an easier way of estimating your BMI. Read off your height and your weight. Where the lines cross in the chart indicates your range of BMI

weight, measured in kilograms, and your height, measured in metres. The recommended BMI is between 20 and 25. To calculate your own BMI, divide your weight by the square of your height. For example, if you weigh 11 stones, that is approximately 70 kg. If you are 5 feet 6 inches tall, that is approximately 168 cm or 1.68 m. Your BMI is the square of your height ($1.68 \times 1.68 = 2.82$) divided into your weight: $70/2.82 = 24.8$. So your BMI is approximately 25 (see page 21).

Stop smoking

Smoking increases the risk of heart disease, fractures and cancers. Women who smoke have a menopause one or two years earlier than non-smokers.

You can do a lot to help your long-term health by making simple lifestyle changes: maintain the correct weight for your height, stop smoking, drink alcohol in moderation, eat plenty of fruit, vegetables and food rich in calcium, and take regular exercise.

Complementary treatments

Many women are concerned about the effects of drugs on their bodies and are keen to find alternative ways to control their symptoms. Acupuncture, aromatherapy, biofeedback, herbalism, homoeopathy, osteopathy, physiotherapy and other treatments may be helpful but there is little research into the benefits and potential risks. It is important to go to qualified therapists. Further information can be obtained from the official organisations representing each of the specialties – see Useful addresses (page 114).

KEEPING HEALTHY

Check your breasts

Self-examination of the breasts is very important. Every woman's breasts are different so it is much easier for her to identify any changes. Research shows that most breast lumps are detected by the woman herself rather than by mass screening programmes. Numerous leaflets are available at the doctor's surgery or pharmacy to show how to check the breasts. Ideally, women should check their breasts every month, at the end of a period as the hormonal changes just before a period swell the breasts and can make it harder to feel any lumps. Go to the doctor if anything unusual or worrying is noticed.

Women aged between 50 and 64 are routinely invited for breast screening every three years, and this may soon be extended to women up to and including the age of 70. Once women reach the upper age limit for routine invitations for breast screening, they are encouraged to continue regular screening by making their own appointment, particularly if they are taking HRT.

Keep up to date with smear tests

Cervical screening or the 'smear test' helps prevent cancer by detecting and treating early abnormalities which, if left untreated, could lead to cancer in a woman's cervix (the neck of the uterus). Early detection and treatment can prevent 80 to 90 per cent of cancers developing. All women between the ages of 25 and 64 are eligible for a free cervical smear test every three to five years.

If you have any tests such as a cervical smear or mammogram, ask how long it is likely to take before you will get the results. If you don't hear within a couple of weeks of this date, contact the clinic or your doctor.

See your doctor if you:

- have any unusual bleeding or very heavy or prolonged bleeding
- notice changes in your usual menstrual pattern

The speculum has two blades, which once opened hold the vaginal walls apart so that the cervix can be seen

View of healthy cervix

Doctor

Patient

Leg support

Bladder

Uterus

Cervix

Speculum (open)

Vagina

Rectum

Cervical screening or the 'smear test' helps prevent cancer by detecting and treating early abnormalities which, if left untreated, could lead to cancer in a woman's cervix.

- have bleeding more than six months after your last period
- bleed after sexual intercourse
- notice any new breast lumps or changes in lumps that have been checked in the past

- have a discharge from your nipple(s)
- notice puckering of your breast skin, like the skin of an orange
- have any concerns or worries about your health

KEY POINTS

✓ Try simple measures and lifestyle changes first

✓ Stop smoking and eat a healthy diet

✓ Maintain a healthy weight

✓ Take regular exercise

✓ Drink alcohol in moderation

✓ Check your breasts regularly

✓ Be sure to attend for routine cervical smears and breast check/mammogram appointments

Replacing the hormones (HRT)

WHAT IS HRT?

Hormone replacement therapy (HRT) does exactly what its name suggests – it replaces the ovarian hormones, oestrogen and progesterone, that are no longer produced when the ovaries cease to function at the time of the menopause.

WHY TAKE HRT?

HRT is the most effective treatment for the symptoms of oestrogen deficiency. The most common symptoms are hot flushes and night sweats but many women also suffer vaginal dryness and urinary frequency and urgency. Women at risk of osteoporosis benefit from HRT, although non-hormonal options are now also available.

HOW LONG HAS HRT BEEN AVAILABLE?

Many women mistakenly believe that HRT is a new invention. In fact, written accounts exist from every era: even the ancient Egyptians sought ways to provide relief. The first documented prescription for HRT was in 1896 when a German gynaecologist gave 'ovarian therapy' to a 23-year-old woman who had had her ovaries removed.

However, early trials of HRT achieved little, because natural oestrogen is poorly absorbed when taken orally. The breakthrough came in the 1930s when attempts at manufacturing synthetic oestrogen were successful. At the same time, natural 'conjugated equine oestrogens', a mixture of several different oestrogens extracted from the urine of pregnant mares, were shown to be effective when taken by mouth. HRT was born and quickly became available commercially. Over the years, further developments have enabled natural human oestrogens to be produced. Most types of HRT available in the UK now contain oestrogen that is structurally indistinguishable from oestrogen produced by the human ovaries.

FEMININE FOREVER?

The 1960s heralded a boom in HRT when Robert Wilson published the highly debated best-seller *Feminine Forever*. He maintained that the menopause was an oestrogen deficiency disease that should be treated with oestrogen to prevent the inevitable 'living decay'. This led to the myth that oestrogen could be used as a panacea for all the effects of ageing.

HEALING OR HARM?

By the mid-1970s doctors had noticed an increase in cancer of the lining of the uterus, or endometrium, in women taking oestrogen. The oestrogen was stimulating growth of the endometrium resulting in the formation of potentially cancerous cells. Fortunately, a simple means to protect the uterus was found – progestogen (synthetic progesterone) was combined with the oestrogen. Progestogen opposes the effect of oestrogen on the endometrium, preventing cancerous changes. Hence an oestrogen/progestogen combination is now generally recommended for women with a uterus whereas women who have had a hysterectomy need take only oestrogen.

Numerous studies followed suggesting that HRT did not just treat symptoms of the menopause, it also prevented the long-term consequences of oestrogen deficiency: osteoporosis, heart attacks and strokes.

Prescription of HRT continued to rise but not everyone was so convinced of the benefits. Some doctors considered that the 'healthy user effect' explained the positive effects of HRT. The 'healthy user effect' suggested that women taking HRT might be more likely to look after themselves in other ways such as not smoking, looking after their diet and taking regular exercise. So these women would be at a lower risk of osteoporosis, heart disease and strokes, whether or not they took HRT.

More recent studies have tried to account for this and consider the overall risks versus benefits of HRT. All the trials have confirmed the benefits of HRT on osteoporosis, and have been consistent in showing an increasing risk of breast cancer associated with duration of use of combined oestrogen and progestogen taken by women who have not had a hysterectomy. In contrast, no increased risk in breast cancer was found in women who had a hysterectomy and were using oestrogen-only therapy. Another finding has been the lack of benefit of HRT on heart disease and strokes.

THE IMPLICATIONS OF RECENT STUDIES ON HRT

Barely a month passes without another headline in the press about HRT. Notably, though, most of the headlines report possible risks rather than benefits.

The major studies to date are the Heart and Estrogen/Progestogen Replacement Study (HERS) (US spelling is estrogen) and the Women's Health Initiative (WHI) study. Both studies have been undertaken in the USA. Half the women in each study were randomly assigned to receive the hormone medication and the other half to receive inactive pills (placebo). Neither the study participants nor the researchers knew who was taking hormones or who was taking placebo. Medical studies with this design are known as randomised, placebo-controlled, double-masked, clinical trials. They are considered to be the 'gold-standard' trial design to demonstrate a cause-and-effect connection between a particular medical condition and treatment. In contrast, observational studies can be misleading. An example is the UK Million Women Study, which claimed that HRT nearly doubles the risk of breast cancer. These results conflict with those from placebo-controlled trials.

Heart and Estrogen/Progestogen Replacement Study

The HERS was designed to look at the effect of HRT on the rate of recurrent heart problems in women who already had heart disease. In all, 2,763 post-menopausal women, with an average age of 67, participated. None of the women had had a hysterectomy. Half of the women were given oestrogen and progestogen every day; the other half took placebo. The study found that taking oestrogen and progestogen for up to four years did not prevent further heart attacks or death from previous heart disease, despite there being a positive effect of HRT on cholesterol. In the first year of the study there was an increased number of heart problems in the women taking active (HRT) medication compared with the inactive (placebo) group. However, after two or more years, the active group had fewer heart problems. This led the investigators to conclude that HRT should not be started by women in order to prevent heart problems. However, they also stated that it might be appropriate for women to continue HRT if they are already taking it when they develop a heart problem. This is because of the possible benefit from longer treatment.

Women's Health Initiative study

The WHI study is a set of clinical trials and an observational study set up by the National Institutes of Health (NIH) in the USA. It was designed to test the risks and benefits of postmenopausal hormone therapy, diet modification, and calcium and vitamin D supplements on heart disease, breast and colorectal cancer, and bone fractures in post-menopausal women. More than 160,000 women aged 50–79 were enrolled as WHI participants between 1993 and 1998.

The hormone trial had two arms: daily oestrogen and progestogen given to women with a uterus and daily oestrogen-only given to women who had had a hysterectomy. The trial was designed primarily to assess the benefit of hormones on the risk of heart disease, because the results of previous studies had suggested that hormones reduced this risk. At the same time, the trial assessed the risk of breast cancer, which was thought to increase with the duration of hormone use.

The oestrogen/progestogen arm was expected to run until 2005 but was stopped in 2002 as a greater than anticipated number of breast cancers occurred in the women taking hormones compared with those taking placebo. The NIH felt that the potential risks of this particular type of HRT in this particular group of women outweighed the benefits. The essential findings were that over 5.2 years of follow-up, women taking HRT had more heart attacks, strokes, blood clots and breast cancers compared with women taking placebo. However, women taking HRT had fewer bone fractures and colorectal cancers.

Similarly, the oestrogen-only arm was stopped early in 2004 because the NIH believed that there were enough data to answer the main study question, and the balance of benefits and risks was not likely to change further. Like the oestrogen/progestogen study, the oestrogen-only study also noted in the active (HRT) group an increased number of strokes during the 6.8 years of follow-up and fewer fractures. In contrast, there were fewer breast cancers, although this benefit was not significantly different from placebo. Nor was there any difference in the number of colorectal cancers or heart attacks between active and placebo treatment.

The reason for these differences will be a major focus of data analyses over the next few years, because there may be reasons other than hormones to account for these findings. For example, certain health factors may be different for women who have had a hysterectomy compared with those who have not.

What do these results mean?

It is very important to be aware that these results apply only to the specific type of HRT used in the studies, the route of delivery, the dose and the type of progestogen – in this case tablets of 0.625 mg conjugated equine oestrogens taken daily with or without 2.5 mg medroxyprogesterone acetate.

Conjugated oral oestrogens derived from the urine of pregnant mares may not have the same effects as human oestrogens or other non-oral routes of oestrogen such as skin patches or gels.

Although the type of HRT used was typical at the time these trials were designed, most HRT we use now contains oestradiol, the same oestrogen produced by human ovaries.

Furthermore, HRT is increasingly being prescribed at lower doses, by non-oral routes and containing different types of progestogens.

Another criticism of the WHI study is that it included women with an average age of 63 – not the typical user, as most women start HRT around the age of 50. Older women will have been deficient of oestrogen for several years and will have a different response to oestrogen from those who are closer to the menopause when they start to take it.

When data from the younger women in the WHI study are analysed, there is actually a reduced risk of heart attacks in this group. In addition, the WHI study and the HERS show that, although there was an increased number of heart attacks in the first year of the trials in the women taking HRT, the risk diminished with time. The authors conclude that long-term use of HRT may actually reduce the risk of heart attacks.

So where does this leave women already taking HRT, or considering starting it? The results of the WHI study can really be applied only to women in their 60s who start conjugated equine oestrogens, with or without medroxyprogesterone acetate.

We know that there are very few risks associated with short-term use of HRT for women starting to take it around age 50 for menopausal symptoms. However, we still don't know the risks and benefits if the same women decide to continue HRT long term, that is, for more than five years. Nor do we really know which is the best type of HRT to take.

All these points are the subjects of ongoing research. In the meantime, the choice of HRT remains individual – each woman has a personal set of risks and benefits. When reading through this book, it might be helpful to note down your own potential risks and benefits to help you consider what is right for you.

HRT: RISKS VS BENEFITS

In deciding whether to take HRT, it is important to consider all the benefits and risks for your own personal situation.

HRT

Risks

- ↑ risk of breast cancer (combined oestrogen/progestrogen)
- ↑ risk of stroke
- ↑ risk of thombosis
- ↑ risk of endometrial cancer (unopposed oestrogen)

Benefits

- ↓ menopausal symptoms
- ↓ risk of fracture
- ↓ risk of colorectal cancer (combined oestrogen/progestrogen)

HRT

RISKS

BENEFITS

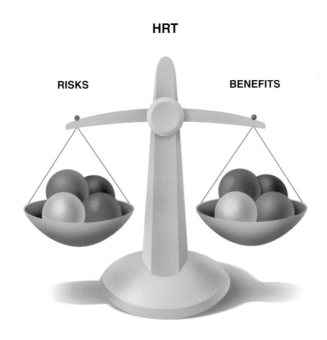

KEY POINTS

✓ HRT aims to restore oestrogen levels using natural oestrogen in doses that mimic the average levels produced during the normal menstrual cycle

✓ HRT is not a panacea for the effects of ageing

✓ Many doctors in the UK recommend non-oral routes of oestradiol, the same oestrogen made naturally by the ovaries

✓ There is still a great deal of research necessary to find the most effective and safest type of HRT

✓ The choice of whether or not to use HRT is individual and should be based on your own balance of potential risks and benefits

The benefits of HRT

HRT can benefit several groups of women. These are considered below.

WOMEN WHO HAVE AN EARLY MENOPAUSE

The average age at menopause is 51, but it can occur in younger women. If you have a menopause under the age of 40, it is recognised as a premature menopause.

Often no cause for a premature menopause is found but it can also be a result of radiotherapy or chemotherapy for cancer, or following surgical removal of the ovaries (oophorectomy). Women who have a hysterectomy but retain their ovaries frequently reach menopause a few years earlier than would otherwise have occurred.

Women who have an untreated premature menopause are at particular risk of developing osteoporosis and heart disease. They are more likely to die at a younger age than women who have the menopause at the usual time.

To reduce these risks, HRT is usually recommended until at least the age of 50. Unlike HRT used beyond the average age at menopause, HRT for a premature menopause is merely replacing hormones that would normally be present. There is no evidence that HRT increases the risk of breast cancer, heart disease or strokes over and above that found in menstruating women with a normally timed menopause. After 50, HRT can be continued if there are reasons to do so and should be reviewed annually.

WOMEN WITH MENOPAUSAL SYMPTOMS

HRT is very effective in relieving the symptoms of the menopause. The lowest dose of oestrogen necessary to control symptoms is recommended. Hot flushes and night sweats usually improve within a few weeks of starting treatment. Vaginal dryness or soreness and urinary urgency and frequency may take longer to respond. Most women using HRT solely for control of menopausal symptoms should not need to take it for more than five years, although longer treatment may be necessary if symptoms recur when HRT is stopped. It is important gradually to reduce HRT over two or three months to assess the return of any symptoms. If HRT is stopped too quickly flushes and sweats will return just because of the sudden drop in hormone levels.

WOMEN AT RISK OF OSTEOPOROSIS

Osteoporosis is a disease in which bones become more fragile and so more likely to break.

Oestrogen plays an important role in building and maintaining bone. Throughout a person's life, old bone breaks down and new bone forms in the skeleton. In childhood and adolescence, new bone is formed faster than old bone is broken down, and the bones become larger, heavier and denser. Women usually have their peak amount of bone around age 35. When oestrogen levels fall following the menopause, the rate of bone loss increases and less new bone is

Periosteum
Strong, dense compact bone
Spongy bone
Periosteum
Thin, weak compact bone
Thin, broken spongy bone
Normal bone
Osteoporotic bone

Changes in osteoporotic bone.

formed. In some women, the bone loss can be so great that the bones become osteoporotic and the risk of fractures increases. About one in three women over the age of 50 fracture a bone as a result of osteoporosis. HRT prevents osteoporosis but needs to be continued for life because bone strength starts to fall when treatment is stopped. Within

Hip fracture.

Wrist fracture.

five years of stopping HRT, the benefit of HRT on bone has been lost. This means that, unless a woman is at particular risk of osteoporosis, the risks of long-term HRT may out-weigh the benefits.

Osteoporosis can be confirmed by measuring bone mineral density using dual energy X-ray absorptiometry (DEXA). Recent advice from the regulatory authorities is that HRT should not be used as a first-line treatment for osteoporosis. However, menopause specialists believe that the balance remains in favour of HRT for women who are at particular risk of osteoporosis. HRT is still recommended for women who are unable to take alternative treatments or for whom other treatments have been unsuccessful.

The table on page 37 shows factors associated with increased

Osteoporotic bone tissue in a vertebra

Loss of height and 'dowager's hump'

Normal bone tissue in a vertebra

Osteoporosis is a common form of bone disease mainly affecting women after the menopause. Hormonal changes lead to a thinning of the interior structure of the bones, making them weaker and more prone to fracture. Weakened vertebrae may become crushed, causing loss of height and severe bending forwards, giving a hunched appearance.

DEXA machine

L1
L2
L3
L4

Monitor image
of lumbar spine

Dual energy X-ray absorptiometry (DEXA).

risk of osteoporosis; the more risk factors you have, the higher your personal risk.

Increased age
The older you are, the greater your risk of fractures.

MAJOR RISK FACTORS FOR OSTEOPOROSIS

- Early menopause
- Increased age
- High alcohol consumption
- Smoking
- Low body mass index
- Family history
- Lack of exercise
- Extended bed rest
- Calcium-deficient diet
- History of infrequent or absent periods
- Certain medical conditions
- Lack of exposure to daylight
- Previous fractures
- Certain racial origins
- Prolonged steroid use
- High caffeine intake

FACTORS PROTECTIVE FOR OSTEOPOROSIS

- Oral contraception use
- High number of pregnancies

High alcohol intake

Following current recommendations, women should stick to a limit of 14 units of alcohol, ideally spread evenly over a week. One unit is equivalent to a small glass of wine, a single measure of spirits or half a pint of beer. If you keep within this limit, it is unlikely that alcohol will be detrimental to your health and may even give some protection against heart disease. Moderate-to-heavy drinking, more than three to five units a day, is associated with an increased fracture risk.

Smoking

Chemicals from tobacco smoke in the bloodstream can affect bones and hasten bone loss.

Low body mass index

How to calculate your body mass index (BMI) is explained in 'Helping yourself' (on page 21). The ideal BMI is between 20 and 25. A BMI of less than 19 is associated with an increased risk of osteoporosis and fractures. A BMI of over 25 indicates an increased risk of high blood pressure, diabetes and heart disease.

Family history

If a blood relative, particularly your mother, has lost height or has fractured a hip or wrist through osteoporosis, it is more likely that you will also fracture a bone.

Lack of exercise

Exercise helps strengthen bones, so if you drive to a sedentary job you are at greater risk of osteoporosis than someone who is on her feet all day. Regular weight-bearing exercise is best for bones, such as brisk walking, aerobics or dancing.

OTHER RISK FACTORS

Extended rest

Bed rest leads to rapid bone loss. If it is necessary to stay in bed for extended periods of time, physiotherapy and simple exercise will help reduce bone loss.

High caffeine intake

Drinking copious cups of coffee or strong tea during the day has been linked to osteoporosis. It is difficult to state a maximum level of intake, although no more than two to four cups a day is generally recommended. Watch for caffeine in other products, particularly canned colas and some health drinks.

Calcium-deficient diet

Adequate amounts of calcium are essential to maintain bone strength. Women need at least 700 to 1,200 mg a day. If you restrict calcium-rich dairy products in your diet, it may be worth boosting your calcium with a supplement.

History of infrequent or absent periods

Amenorrhoea (lack of menstrual periods) for longer than one year is associated with insufficient oestrogen to maintain a normal menstrual cycle. Oestrogen deficiency is the result. Long periods of dieting and anorexia nervosa are common causes in young women. Young gymnasts or marathon runners are also at risk. Some treatments for endometriosis (when the uterine lining is found in tissues outside the uterus) stimulate a temporary menopause by switching off the production of oestrogen. All these situations can increase the risk of oestrogen deficiency symptoms and diseases.

Certain medical conditions

An overactive thyroid increases the resting metabolic rate, speeding up the normal process of bone formation and breakdown, which can lead to osteoporosis. Other medical conditions associated with an increased risk of osteoporosis include Cushing's disease, inflammatory bowel disease, chronic liver disease, coeliac disease and rheumatoid arthritis.

Lack of daylight

Elderly women often stay indoors and get little sunlight on their skin. In certain cultures women are heavily covered in dark clothing and, particularly if they live in Europe, minimal daylight reaches their skin. Sunlight is very important because it stimulates the production of vitamin D in the skin. Vitamin D aids the absorption of calcium from food, helping bones to stay strong and healthy. Only 10 to 15 minutes of sun exposure at least twice a week to the face, arms, hands, or back, without sunscreen, is usually sufficient to provide adequate vitamin D.

Previous fractures

Previous fractures suggest existing osteoporosis, increasing the likelihood of further broken bones.

Certain racial origins

Women of African–Caribbean racial origin achieve a 10 per cent greater peak bone mass than women of European extraction, hence the latter population are at greater risk of osteoporosis.

Prolonged steroid use

Prolonged use of oral steroids, over five milligrams each day for more than three months, is linked to osteoporosis. Steroids are usually prescribed for conditions such as severe asthma or other autoimmune diseases. In these conditions the body's protective mechanisms are disrupted and normal tissue is seen as a foreign body that should be destroyed.

Short-term courses of steroids, taken for one or two weeks, are not associated with increased risks unless repeated frequently. If you are on long-term steroid therapy, speak to your doctor to discuss alternative therapy and ways that you can prevent osteoporosis developing.

PROTECTIVE FACTORS
Oral contraceptive use
Studies have shown a lower risk of fractures in women who have taken combined oral contraceptives for five years or more during their 30s or 40s (see pages 99–100).

High number of pregnancies
Research shows an increase in bone density with increasing parity (the number of pregnancies a woman delivers past 28 weeks.) The positive effect on bone density has been seen in both pre- and post-menopausal women. One study concluded that women with three or more children had a 30–40 per cent reduction in hip fracture risk when compared with nulliparous women (those who have never given birth).

OSTEOPOROSIS: THE ALTERNATIVES TO HRT
For a fuller explanation of these treatments see the Family Doctor book *Understanding Osteoporosis*.

First-line treatments
Bisphosphonates are a group of medicines that include alendronate (brand or proprietary name Fosamax) and risedronate (proprietary name Actonel) which are available on prescription. These are the most commonly used medicines to treat osteoporosis and prevent bone loss. They are the preferred choice for women in their 60s who need treatment. Long-term safety over 20 years is not known and some research suggests that, although they may increase the amount of bone, the new bone formed is not as strong as bone formed by oestrogens. Hence many specialists recommend that younger women at risk of osteoporosis would gain most benefit from long-term treatment with HRT.

Second-line treatments
Other drugs available on prescription include bisphosphonate etidronate (Didronel), calcitonin (Miacalcic) and raloxifene (Evista).

Calcitonin is a hormone that slows down bone loss and increases the density of the spinal bone. However, the effects of calcitonin on fracture risk remain unclear. Raloxifene belongs to a relatively new group of drugs known as selective oestrogen receptor modulators, or SERMs. These drugs are

CALCIUM SUPPLEMENTS

Calcium supplement	Dose (milligrams)	Formulation
Adcal	600	Chewable tablets
Calcium gluconate	53	Tablet
Calcium lactate	39	Tablet
Cacit	500	Effervescent tablets
Calcichew	500	Chewable tablets
Calcichew Forte	1,000	Chewable tablets
Calcium-500	500	Tablet
Calcium-Sandoz	108	Syrup
Ossopan	178	Tablet
Ossopan	712	Granules
Ostram	1,200	Powder
Sandocal	400	Effervescent tablets
Sandocal 1000	1,000	Effervescent tablets

Amounts of calcium are shown per tablet or dose.

COMBINED CALCIUM AND VITAMIN D PREPARATIONS

Preparation	Vitamin D (IU/dose)	Calcium (mg/dose)	Formulation
Calcium and vitamin D	400	97	Chewable tablet
Adcal-D$_3$	400	600	Chewable tablet
Cacit D$_3$	440	500	Granules
Calceos	400	500	Chewable tablet
Calcichew D$_3$	200	500	Chewable tablet
Calcichew D$_3$ Forte	400	500	Chewable tablet
Calfovit D$_3$	800	1,200	Powder

DRUGS FOR OSTEOPOROSIS

Calcitonin

Miacalcic (Novartis)
- calcitonin 200 IU per spray (nasal spray)

Vitamin D analogue

Rocaltrol (Roche)
- calcitriol 0.25 micrograms (capsules)
- calcitriol 0.5 micrograms (capsules)

Bisphosphonate/calcium

Didronel PMO (Proctor & Gamble)
- etridonate disodium 400 mg (tablets)
- calcium carbonate 1,250 mg (effervescent tablets)

Bisphosphonate

Actonel (Procter & Gamble/Aventis)
- risedronate sodium 5 mg (tablets)
OR
Actonel Once a Week (Procter & Gamble/Aventis)
- risedronate sodium 35 mg (tablets)
Fosomax (MSD)
- alendronate sodium (equivalent to 5 mg alendronic acid) (tablets)
OR
- alendronate sodium (equivalent to 10 mg alendronic acid) (tablets)
OR
Fosomax Once Weekly (MSD)
- alendronate sodium (tablets)

Selective oestrogen receptor modulator (SERM)

Evista (Lilly)
- raloxifene hydrochloride 60 mg (tablets)

Parathyroid hormone

Forsteo (Lilly)
- teriperatide 20 micrograms per ml in a 3-ml prefilled pen for subcutaneous injection

Strontium

Protelos (Serner)
- Strontium ranelate 2 g granules

not oestrogens but have oestrogen-like effects on bone, increasing bone mass and reducing the risk of spinal fractures.

Teriparatide (Forsteo), a drug identical to human parathyroid hormone, is occasionally used but has to be given by daily injection under the skin of the thigh or abdomen. Unlike the bisphosphonates, teriparatide stimulates bone formation rather than just slowing down the rate at which bone is lost.

Strontium ranelate also increases bone formation as well as preventing bone loss. It is taken once daily at bedtime, dissolved in water.

OTHER BENEFITS OF HRT

Arthritis

Increasing evidence suggests that HRT reduces the symptoms of arthritis, although it is not licensed (see Glossary, page 111) for this indication. This is true for both osteoarthritis and rheumatoid arthritis. Although HRT does not reverse the process of these conditions, it is a useful adjunct to conventional therapy and is worth discussing with your GP or specialist.

Colorectal cancer

The incidence of colorectal cancer is rising. Between 1971 and 1997 in the UK the total number of cases increased by 42 per cent, from 20,400 to 28,900. In 2003, over 30,000 people in the UK were diagnosed with this condition. This makes colorectal cancer the second most common cancer that affects women (after breast cancer). Recent studies suggest that HRT may reduce the risk of developing colorectal cancer by about one-third.

KEY POINTS

✓ HRT is of particular benefit to women who have a premature menopause as these women are at high risk of osteoporosis in later life

✓ For women who have had a premature menopause, if HRT is taken until 51 – the average age at menopause – there is no evidence of increased risks associated with its use

✓ HRT is the most effective treatment for menopausal symptoms

✓ HRT is one of several treatments that are effective for osteoporosis

✓ HRT has been shown to reduce the risk of colorectal cancer and to improve symptoms of arthritis

The risks of HRT

Although HRT can offer many benefits, for some women it can carry unacceptable potential risks. When deciding whether or not HRT is right for you, you must consider the balance between risks and benefits.

The main potential risks that have been identified are breast cancer, blood clots in the veins (venous thrombosis) and arteries (heart attacks and strokes), and cancer of the lining of the uterus (endometrium), although the last can be prevented by the addition of progestogen. It is important to understand these risks and put them into perspective – most women taking HRT do not experience any of these problems as a direct result of taking the hormones. Furthermore, other risk factors are often more important than HRT – particularly smoking or being very overweight – in creating these problems.

BREAST CANCER
Women starting HRT before the age of 50 for a premature menopause do not have an increased risk of breast cancer. This indicates that it is the duration of lifetime exposure to oestrogen that is the relevant factor in causing breast cancer.

So those women who have a late natural menopause or take HRT beyond the age of 50 are at higher risk of developing breast cancer than women who have a menopause at the more usual time (51) because they will have had a greater lifetime exposure to oestrogen. After stopping HRT the risk of breast cancer gradually returns to the same level as for women who have never taken HRT. By five years after stopping HRT, there is no difference in risk between women who have taken HRT and women who have never taken HRT.

Breast cancer is not uncommon

in women in later life even when not using HRT – about 1 in 15 (67 in 1,000) older women will develop breast cancer before they reach the age of 70. Studies show that HRT started after the menopause must be taken for at least five years before the risk of breast cancer increases.

Recent studies suggest that the risks of breast cancer are associated with combined oestrogen/progestogen HRT, necessary for women who have not had a hysterectomy, whereas oestrogen-only HRT appears not to increase risk. For example, the WHI study between 1993 and 1998 showed that, for women aged between 50 and 79, there were around 30 cases of breast cancer each year for every 10,000 women who were not taking HRT. In comparison, for every 10,000 women taking HRT there were:

- about eight **extra** cases of breast cancer each year in women taking conjugated equine oestrogen combined with medroxyprogesterone acetate (combined oestrogen/progestogen HRT)
- about seven **fewer** cases of breast cancer each year in women taking conjugated equine oestrogen (oestrogen-only HRT).

Most women are now given different types of HRT to those used in the studies and we do not know whether or not the findings can be extended to these newer types of HRT. Since then natural oestradiol has become available and is most commonly used. Also, an increasing number of women use non-oral HRT such as patches and gels, which enables a smaller dose to be given with the same effect as a higher dose of tablets. This is because, when a tablet is swallowed, the hormones are absorbed in the gut and have to pass through the liver before they reach the bloodstream. Once in the bloodstream, the hormones can be circulated all around the body. However, the liver breaks down hormones, so not all the dose of hormones swallowed actually reaches the blood. In contrast, patches and gels enable hormones to pass through the skin, directly into the bloodstream.

In the light of these results, however, women who haven't had a hysterectomy may be tempted to take oestrogen-only HRT, but it must be remembered that progestogen is necessary to protect against endometrial cancer (see page 27).

The risk of developing breast cancer appears to be related to the number of years of exposure to oestrogen and progestogen. Early onset of menstruation before the age of 12 years is associated with about a twofold increase in the risk of breast cancer.

Women who have premature

NON-HRT RISK FACTORS FOR BREAST CANCER

- Family history
- Older age at birth of first child
- Late menopause
- Early menarche (age at first period)
- Postmenopausal obesity
- Alcohol – more than two to three units/day

menopause will have a reduction in the risk of developing breast cancer. These women typically may have a 50 per cent reduction in the risk of breast cancer, but are at much higher risk for heart disease and osteoporosis.

A first full-term pregnancy after age 30 is associated with a 50 per cent increased risk of breast cancer compared with women who have their children before this age.

The role of the protective effect of breast-feeding on breast cancer is not very clear, but there is some evidence to suggest that this may be the case.

A high body mass index (BMI), over 30, also increases the risk of breast cancer by 50 per cent compared with women with a normal BMI of 25 or lower.

Current medical research suggests that there may be an inherited risk of breast cancer. A family history of breast cancer in a close relative usually indicates a greater personal risk but there is no

evidence to show that using HRT further increases the risk. However, if you are at high risk of breast cancer and have a low risk of osteoporosis and minimal menopausal symptoms, there is little advantage in taking HRT. If you are experiencing marked flushes and sweats, and have no risk factors for breast cancer, HRT might be a good choice for you.

HRT for women treated for breast cancer

Although HRT is increasingly considered to be an effective option for severe flushes and sweats resulting from the treatment of breast cancer, its use is controversial and the results of studies are conflicting. However, HRT is offered in several specialist breast cancer centres where the doctors have more experience of using HRT in these circumstances. Alternative approaches to debilitating menopausal symptoms in women treated for breast cancer include vaginal oestrogen (creams,

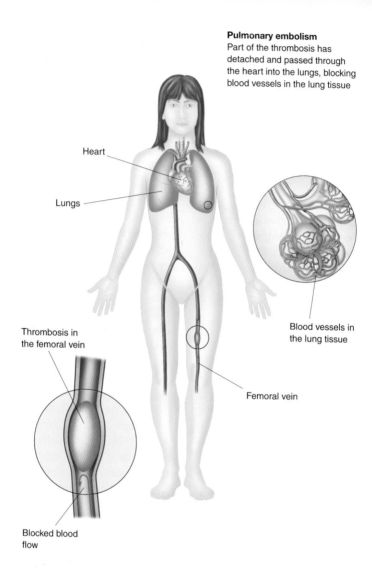

Pulmonary embolism
Part of the thrombosis has detached and passed through the heart into the lungs, blocking blood vessels in the lung tissue

Heart

Lungs

Blood vessels in the lung tissue

Thrombosis in the femoral vein

Femoral vein

Blocked blood flow

Deep vein thrombosis is a condition in which a blood clot forms in a large vein, usually in the leg. There is a risk that the clot may travel through the heart and become lodged in another part of the body, for instance a blood vessel supplying the lungs, which can be fatal.

pessaries, tablets and rings) to help vaginal dryness. For hot flushes and sweats, non-hormonal treatments such as selective serotonin reuptake inhibitors (SSRIs – antidepressants) may help (see page 97).

VENOUS THROMBOSIS

Increasing age is the main risk for venous thrombosis (blood clots in veins). However, research suggests that women using HRT are more likely to develop venous thrombosis than women of a similar age who are not using HRT, especially in the first year of use. About three per 1,000 women in their 50s who do not use HRT are likely to have a venous thrombosis in any five-year period compared with seven per 1,000 women of the same age who take HRT.

By the time they reach their 60s, the risk in non-users increases to eight per 1,000 women in a five-year period compared with 17 per 1,000 women taking HRT. However, published data suggest that non-oral HRT such as patches and gels is less likely to increase the risk of ven-ous thrombosis than HRT tablets.

If you have multiple risk factors for venous thrombosis (see below), HRT is probably best avoided. If you have major surgery and will be off your feet for a while, you will probably be given drugs to help prevent blood clots. Some doctors advise stopping HRT four to six weeks before major surgery. You can usually start HRT again once you are fully mobile.

If you or a close relative has had an unexplained venous thrombosis under the age of 45, you may need to have a blood test to check your blood clotting before you can take HRT. This can identify those women who have a genetic risk factor for venous thrombosis, the most common of which is known as factor V Leiden. This genetic condition affects around five per cent of the population and causes an increased tendency for blood to clot. People carrying the factor V Leiden gene have a five times greater risk of developing a blood clot than the rest of the population.

NON-HRT RISK FACTORS FOR VENOUS THROMBOSIS

- Severe varicose veins
- Obesity
- Increased age
- Inactivity
- Diabetes
- High blood pressure

HEART ATTACKS AND STROKES

It is quite rare for a woman to suffer a heart attack or a stroke before the menopause; the incidence starts to rise in postmenopausal women. Heart disease is now recognised as the leading cause of early death in women, more significant than any type of cancer. Twenty per cent of postmenopausal women are at risk of stroke, with an eight per cent chance of death. Likewise, postmenopausal women have a 46 per cent chance of developing coronary heart disease at some point with a one in three chance of it causing death.

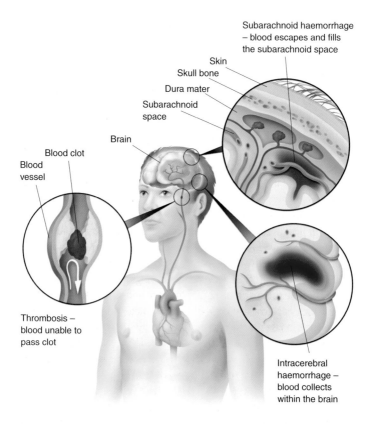

Subarachnoid haemorrhage – blood escapes and fills the subarachnoid space

Skin

Skull bone

Dura mater

Subarachnoid space

Brain

Blood clot

Blood vessel

Thrombosis – blood unable to pass clot

Intracerebral haemorrhage – blood collects within the brain

The most common cause of a stroke is a thrombosis – when a blood vessel supplying the brain becomes blocked with a blood clot. The second most common cause of a stroke is a brain haemorrhage, of which there are two types; both involve a blood vessel bursting inside the head.

With respect to stroke, about three out of 1,000 women in their 50s not using HRT can expect to have a stroke in any 5-year period. For women of a similar age who use HRT for 5 years, the figure rises to 4 per 1,000. The risk rises with age, so the risk in non-HRT users in their 60s is 11 per 1,000 in any 5-year period compared with 15 per 1,000 women of the same age using HRT.

Until recently, it was always thought that HRT protected against heart disease and strokes. This was based on observational studies, comparing HRT users with non-users. The WHI study compared postmenopausal women taking conjugated oestrogen and medroxy-progesterone acetate against women taking inactive treatment. The results suggested that the risk of heart disease was increased in the first year of use. However, the average age of women starting HRT in the study was 63 – much older than women in the observational studies, most of which looked at women starting HRT around the age of 50. The WHI study further showed that, when HRT was continued, there was a significant trend to reduced risk of heart disease, that is, continuing HRT reduced the risk of heart disease.

Furthermore, when the age of women in the WHI study was considered, the women who were between 50 and 59 when they started the study actually had an overall 50 per cent reduction in the risk of heart disease. These findings could be explained by the fact that oestrogen increases blood clotting, increasing the risk of stroke and heart attacks but, in the long term, can prevent a build-up of athero-sclerosis in the blood vessels, reducing the risk of stroke and heart attacks.

If HRT is started in women who are used to having oestrogen in the body, as are women starting HRT around the age of 50, they will be less susceptible to the clotting effects of oestrogen and more likely to benefit from the long-term effects to protect against athero-sclerosis. Older women starting HRT after years of oestrogen de-ficiency will already have developed atherosclerosis and may be more susceptible to the effect of oestrogen on blood clotting.

There are no data yet for other types of HRT which may have a different effect. What is needed is a study of different types of HRT started by women aged between 45 and 56. However, until such studies are undertaken, HRT should not be started to prevent further heart attacks in women who have already had a heart attack.

If you have had angina, a heart attack or stroke in the past, you should see your doctor to discuss the possible benefits and risks of

THE PROCESS OF ATHEROSCLEROSIS

Atherosclerosis, atheroma and hardening of the arteries are all the same thing – the process leading to the blockage or weakening of arteries.

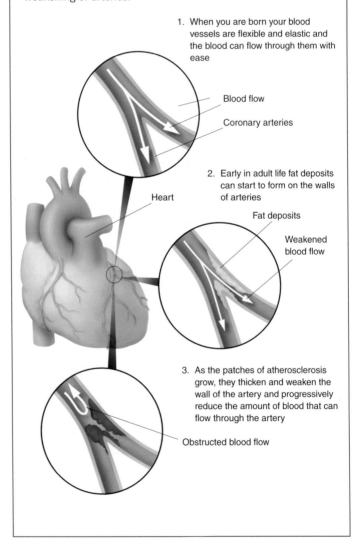

1. When you are born your blood vessels are flexible and elastic and the blood can flow through them with ease

Blood flow

Coronary arteries

Heart

2. Early in adult life fat deposits can start to form on the walls of arteries

Fat deposits

Weakened blood flow

3. As the patches of atherosclerosis grow, they thicken and weaken the wall of the artery and progressively reduce the amount of blood that can flow through the artery

Obstructed blood flow

- High blood pressure
- High cholesterol
- Smoking
- Previous heart attack or stroke
- Irregular heart beat (atrial fibrillation)
- Diabetes
- Obesity
- Personality – people who are competitive and easily stressed are more likely to develop heart disease than people who are laid back about life

HRT for you. However, if you are already taking HRT when you have your first heart attack or stroke, there is probably no reason to stop HRT because continuing treatment may reduce your long-term risk of a repeat event.

CANCER OF THE UTERUS

Around 8 per 100,000 women a year over age 50 who are not using HRT develop cancer of the lining of the uterus (endometrial cancer). Women taking 'unopposed' oestrogen-only HRT for five years have a sixfold increased risk. A breakthrough in research showed that 'opposing' the oestrogen by adding progestogen reduced this risk. With combined oestrogen/progestogen HRT, the risk of endometrial cancer is at least the same as for non-HRT users, if not lower.

OVARIAN CANCER

There appears to be a small increase in the risk of ovarian cancer in women using oestrogen-only HRT for more than five years. The background risk in non-users aged 50 to 69 is 9 per 1,000 women, which rises to 10 per 1,000 women after 5 years' use of oestrogen-only HRT and to 12 per 1,000 women after 10 years of HRT. The effect of long-term combined oestrogen/progestogen HRT on ovarian cancer has not yet been studied.

KEY POINTS

✓ The potential risks of HRT use include breast and endometrial cancer, venous thrombosis and stroke

✓ Use of conjugated equine oestrogens alone does not appear to be associated with an increased risk of breast cancer

✓ HRT containing conjugated equine oestrogens combined with medroxyprogesterone acetate is associated with an increased risk of breast cancer

✓ The risk of breast cancer declines after stopping HRT and, by five years, is the same as if you have never taken it

✓ Taking HRT increases your risk of venous thrombosis, especially in the first year of use

✓ HRT started at the time of the menopause may reduce the long-term risk of heart disease

✓ The potential risks associated with HRT use are smaller than the health risks associated with smoking or being very overweight

Different types of HRT

Hormone replacement therapy (HRT) is available only on prescription. There are numerous different brands of HRT marketed, some containing both oestrogen and progestogen, some containing oestrogen only, in a variety of preparations.

OESTROGEN PREPARATIONS

Oestrogens used in HRT are either natural or synthetic. Both produce effects similar to the oestrogens produced by the ovaries. Natural oestrogens are similar in chemical structure to the oestrogens produced by the ovaries whereas synthetic ones have a different structure. Oestradiol, oestrone and oestriol are natural human ovarian oestrogens. Equilin and 17-alpha-dihydroequilin are natural equine oestrogens derived from the urine of pregnant mares. Dienoestrol, ethinyloestradiol and mestranol are synthetic oestrogens.

Natural oestrogens, both human and equine, are preferred for HRT because they have fewer side effects. Synthetic oestrogens are more potent and so are favoured for contraception because they effectively suppress ovulation. Oestrogens are available for HRT in various forms. For systemic absorption, which means circulating in the bloodstream to all the tissues in the body, they come as tablets, patches, implants and gels, and in a vaginal ring. To apply just to your vagina (local vaginal application) you can get creams, pessaries, tablets and a vaginal ring.

THE DIFFERENT TYPES OF OESTROGEN AND PROGESTOGEN PREPARATIONS

Although tablets are the most common form in which oestrogen and progestogen preparations are supplied, HRT also comes in a variety of other forms. Systemic hormones circulate throughout the body, whereas local vaginal oestrogens treat only vaginal symptoms.

Oestrogen	Progestogen
Systemic	*Systemic*
• Tablets	• Tablets
• Patches	• Patches (combined with oestrogen)
• Implant	
• Gels	*Intrauterine*
• Nasal spray	• Levonorgestrel
• Vaginal ring	intrauterine system (IUS)
Vaginal (local)	*Vaginal (local)*
• Creams	• Gel
• Pessary	• Pessary
• Ring	
• Tablet	

PROGESTOGEN PREPARATIONS

Progesterone is also produced by the ovaries, but it is very unstable in tablet form and it also has a very sedative effect (makes you sleepy). To be effective, natural progesterone tablets must be taken several times a day. Natural progesterone is also available as a vaginal gel or pessary (inserted into the vagina) and suppository (inserted into the back passage), which enables the hormone to be absorbed into the bloodstream through the walls of the vagina or rectum. However, they can be very messy to use.

For convenience, synthetic forms of progesterone are used in HRT, called progestogens. These have similar effects to natural progesterone but are available as oral tablets that can be taken once a day or combined with oestrogen in patches. Oestrogen combined with cyclical progestogen is the HRT most women use if they start HRT before, or shortly after, the menopause. Oestrogen is taken continuously, without a break. A monthly course of progestogen lasting 10 to 14 days mimics the natural hormone cycle in which progesterone is produced for the last 14 days of the cycle, following ovulation. As in the natural menstrual cycle, when the course of progesterone or progestogen is stopped, 'withdrawal' of the hormone results in menstrual bleeding, or a 'period'.

Most women who have gone through the menopause do not wish to return to monthly periods. To avoid this, a combination of oestrogen and progestogen is taken daily. Taking both hormones together prevents any thickening of the uterine lining, making a withdrawal bleed unnecessary while providing protection against endometrial cancer.

ORAL TABLETS

Oestrogen

HRT is most commonly prescribed as tablets. If you have had a hysterectomy, only oestrogen treatment is necessary, because you do not need to take progestogen with the oestrogen to protect your uterus. You should take the tablets every day, without a break, at about the same time each day.

Progestogen

If your periods have not stopped and you have not had a hyster-ectomy, you need to take a course of progestogen every month, for about 10 to 14 days, in order to mimic the natural menstrual cycle. This is usually available in calendar packs, the progestogen combined with oestrogen, so that you do not have to work out when to take them. From around the age of 55 when most women have completely stopped their periods, it is possible to take progestogens together with oestrogen every day – a period-free preparation.

For women who want to take progestogen with their own choice of oestrogen, they are also available separately. If used this way, many doctors recommend that women take the progestogen for the first 10 to 14 days of every calendar month, for instance starting 1 March, 1 April and so on. This has the advantage that the type and dose of oestrogen and progestogen can be adjusted more easily than standard packs. A withdrawal bleed or period should start around the middle of each month, which makes it easy for the doctor to assess if there is any irregular bleeding that may need further investigation.

Women whose last natural period was more than one year ago can take the same dose of progestogen continuously every day.

Advantages of tablets

Most people find tablets easy to take and their effects are quickly reversed if they decide to discontinue treatment (see pages 81–83 for section on stopping HRT).

Disadvantages of tablets

It is not always easy to remember to take tablets every day, and even more difficult to remember when people are away from home. Missing a tablet can trigger fluctuations in hormone levels and irregular bleeding.

It is necessary to take much higher doses of hormones by mouth to allow for huge losses because the hormones are absorbed from the gut and pass through the liver where they are usually broken down and excreted from the body. Such doses can increase side effects. Nausea is more common with tablets than with other routes but can be minimised by taking the tablet with food or at bedtime. Rarely, oral oestrogen is so poorly absorbed that menopausal symptoms are not controlled and an alternative route of HRT administration is recommended.

SKIN PATCHES

Oestrogen

Skin patches provide a means of delivering the hormones directly to the bloodstream through the skin, bypassing the liver. Patches are applied once or twice weekly, depending on the brand. The newer 'matrix' patches, which look just like a thin sheet of plastic, are generally well tolerated. The older-style 'reservoir' patches containing alcohol, which are thicker than the matrix patches and have a round 'reservoir' in the centre of the patch, can cause skin irritation.

To use patches, remove the backing sheet and stick onto clean, dry skin, free from talcum powder, bath oils or body cream. The best site is the upper buttock. Press the patch firmly on your skin for about 10 seconds, then run your fingers around the edges to seal it.

You can keep the patch on when you have a bath or go swimming, although it can be removed temporarily for half an hour or so if you prefer – keep the backing sheet to stick the patch on to until you need it again. Cover the patch when sunbathing and remove it if you are using a sunbed to avoid the sun irritating the skin around the patch. When replacing patches, change the site, for example alternate buttocks, so that you are not sticking the patch in the same place each time as the skin can become red and sore underneath it.

Oestrogen/progestogen combinations

Patches are available that produce a monthly bleed. As with the tablets, they are packaged so that ones containing both oestrogen and pro-gestogen are used for the first two weeks and oestrogen-only patches for the second two weeks.

Postmenopausal women who do not want periods can use combined oestrogen/progestogen patches continuously.

Advantages of patches

Unlike tablets, hormones from patches do not pass through the stomach and liver first, so the dose can be lower, reducing side effects. The hormone levels are also much more constant with patches than with tablets. There are several different strengths available.

Disadvantages of patches

The main disadvantage is that there are not yet many varieties available. At present there is only one dose strength of a combined patch with no choice of the type of oestrogen and progestogen, so adjusting the dose can be difficult.

Occasionally, patches do not stick very well, particularly in hot, sticky weather, but this can easily be remedied by covering the patch with two-inch surgical tape.

Even if a different site is used

Hormones are absorbed through the skin below the patch and into the blood vessels

Skin

Hormones

Blood vessel

Skin-patch containing hormones

Skin patches deliver hormones directly to the bloodstream through the skin. As they do not pass through the stomach and liver first, as tablets do, the required dose is much lower, thus reducing the side effects.

each time as recommended, it is normal for the skin underneath the patch to redden. However, a few women develop a severe skin reaction that prohibits further use. Switching to a different brand of patch can occasionally help.

GEL

Oestrogen, but not progestogen, is available as a gel and is becoming an increasingly popular method of taking HRT. The gel is applied daily to the arms and shoulders, or thighs, and absorbed through the skin into the bloodstream.

Advantages of gel

Many women find a gel convenient and easy to use, with few side effects. Unlike some oestrogen patches, skin irritation is rarely a problem. The dose is easy to change, balanced against symptoms.

Disadvantages of gel

Some women worry that they are not applying the gel to the correct amount of skin. On a practical note, it is easiest just to apply the gel to the upper thighs, like a skin cream, without worrying too much about how much skin is covered. The gel dries quickly and it is only necessary to wait five minutes at most before dressing. Avoid using other skin products or washing the area for an hour after application. Unless the woman has had a hysterectomy, additional progestogen is necessary.

NASAL SPRAY

This relatively new route for oestrogen assimilation works in a different way to other forms of HRT. It is sprayed into the nostrils and is rapidly absorbed through the lining of the nasal passage, delivering a pulse of oestrogen into the bloodstream.

Advantages of nasal spray

Some studies suggest that this method is associated with fewer side effects than other routes of delivery.

Disadvantages of nasal spray

Surges of oestrogen may aggravate conditions such as migraine, which benefit from constant oestrogen levels. Unless the woman has had a hysterectomy, additional progestogen is necessary.

SYSTEMIC VAGINAL RING

A new ring has been developed for insertion into the upper third of the vagina, enabling oestrogen to be absorbed through the lining of the vagina into the bloodstream. This will also effectively treat hot flushes and sweats. It lasts for three months of continuous use before it needs to be replaced.

Advantages of vaginal ring

The main advantages are that it is easy to use with few side effects. It can be removed for intercourse, although this is not necessary. It should be rinsed in lukewarm water before being re-inserted.

Disadvantages of vaginal ring

Some women note initial discomfort, although this usually settles with time. The ring may become dislodged when coughing or straining. Unless the woman has had a hysterectomy, additional progestogen is necessary.

IMPLANTS

Oestrogen

Small pellets of oestrogen, inserted into the fat under the skin of the lower abdomen or buttock, typically last for about six months. The downside is that if the woman decides to stop HRT, they cannot easily be removed. Insertion is a simple procedure that can be done at the local surgery or in the hospital outpatient department. An injection of a local anaesthetic is given to numb the skin before a small cut is made. After the implant is inserted, the wound is closed

Implant insertion device

Patient

Needle

Oestrogen pellet

Skin

Fat layer

Oestrogen pellet is inserted under the skin into the layer of fat

Oestrogen implantation is a simple procedure involving a local anaesthetic, a small cut in the lower abdomen and the insertion of an oestrogen pellet into the layer of fat under the skin. The wound is then closed with a stitch or a piece of tape.

with a stitch or small strips of sticky tape (Steri-Strips).

Testosterone

Testosterone is the main male hormone, although the ovaries produce small amounts. The precise role of testosterone in women is unclear, although there is evidence that low testosterone levels can adversely affect mood, energy and libido. Although adequate oestrogen replacement often resolves these symptoms, testosterone implants are sometimes recommended for women with loss of sexual desire, particularly if they have had their ovaries removed and cannot produce testosterone themselves.

Advantages of implants

The advantage of implants is that, once inserted, you can forget about HRT for at least six months. The implants dissolve slowly and provide constant levels of hormone. Implants produce the highest levels of oestrogen of all forms of HRT, with greatest effect on bone density.

Disadvantages of implants

Minor surgery is needed every six months. Although the pellets usually dissolve completely within about six months, you are often left with lumps of fibrous tissue under the skin. You will also have small scars where the implants were inserted. The main disadvantage is that, if this method does not suit you, it is virtually impossible to remove the pellet once implanted.

An occasional problem is that the implants last increasingly shorter periods of time after each insertion, so that menopausal symptoms return only two or three months after the last implant. Paradoxically, if oestrogen levels are measured, they are very high and it seems as if these women have developed some immunity to the effects of the implant. This phenomenon is known as 'tachyphylaxis' and seems to occur only with implants. Unfortunately, the only way to treat this is to withhold further implants until the oestrogen levels fall to within the normal range. Tachyphylaxis can usually be avoided by measuring oestrogen levels before each implant is inserted to ensure that no more than the necessary dose is given. Many doctors will not insert a new implant without knowing the oestrogen levels at the time of insertion.

Implants are rarely used in women who have not had a hysterectomy because the sustained effect of oestrogen on the endometrium means that it is imperative that progestogen is taken regularly until the oestrogen is completely used up. This may be up to a couple of years after the final implant. This can be a problem for women who experience unwanted side effects of progestogen.

VAGINAL (LOCAL) OESTROGEN

Vaginal creams and pessaries are useful for women who have mostly vaginal symptoms. They are simple and easy to use but can be a bit messy. Vaginal tablets are a more convenient option. All are placed directly into the vagina.

Advantages of local oestrogen
Used correctly there is little risk associated with them. They are extremely useful for women with few symptoms other than a dry vagina or bladder problems. They can be used in addition to standard HRT regimens if vaginal dryness is a continuing problem, although a check with a doctor must be made to exclude non-hormonal causes.

Disadvantages of local oestrogen
Creams and pessaries can be messy. Oestrogen tablets, which come with an applicator ensuring that the oestrogen is placed high in the vagina, and a vaginal ring, are alternative options.

Use them strictly as prescribed because some types of local oestrogen don't just act locally but are absorbed into the bloodstream. In this case, unless the woman has had a hysterectomy, it may be necessary to take additional pro-gestogen. A doctor can advise about the need for this.

OTHER FORMS OF PROGESTOGEN

Natural progesterone
Natural progesterone, structurally the same as progesterone from the ovaries, is available as a vaginal gel. It is generally used every other day for the last 12 days of the cycle to stimulate a withdrawal bleed. In some clinical trials it has been used twice weekly together with oestrogen as part of a continuous combined regimen.

Rectal or vaginal suppositories of natural progesterone are sometimes used for women experiencing bad side effects from progestogen, but doctors rarely prescribe these because they are not licensed (see Glossary, page 111) for HRT.

Natural progesterone creams can be purchased from health-food shops. Used alone, these can alleviate some menopausal symptoms. However, they should not be used as the progestogen component of combined HRT because they do not provide adequate endometrial protection.

Levonorgestrel intrauterine system
The levonorgestrel intrauterine system, or IUS (proprietary name Mirena), is a highly effective contraceptive. It has a reservoir of the

PROGESTOGEN PREPARATIONS

In place of a combined oestrogen/progestogen preparation, the doctor may prescribe one of the oestrogen-only preparations previously listed, together with any of the following progestogen preparations.

Tablets

Duphaston-HRT (Solvay)
- dydrogesterone 10 mg

Micronor-HRT (Janssen-Cilag)
- norethisterone 1 mg

Provera (Pharmacia)
- medroxyprogesterone acetate 2.5 mg, 5 mg or 10 mg

Suppositories/pessaries

Cyclogest (Shire)
- progesterone 200 mg or 400 mg by vagina or rectum

Vaginal gel

Crinone (Serono)
- progesterone 8% (not licensed for HRT)

Intrauterine

Mirena (Schering)
- Levonorgestrel 52 mg (20 mg per 24 hours)

progestogen levonorgestrel, which is slowly released directly into the uterus, keeping the lining of the uterus thin so that there is no build-up of lining to be shed as a 'period'.

Side effects are much lower than with other progestogens and the contraceptive effect can be an advantage for women whose periods have not yet stopped. The main disadvantage is irregular bleeding but, for most women, periods stop completely.

OTHER PRESCRIPTION TREATMENTS
Tibolone

Tibolone (Livial) is a synthetic preparation of a type known as a selective tissue oestrogenic activity regulator (STEAR). It is derived from plant sources and combines the

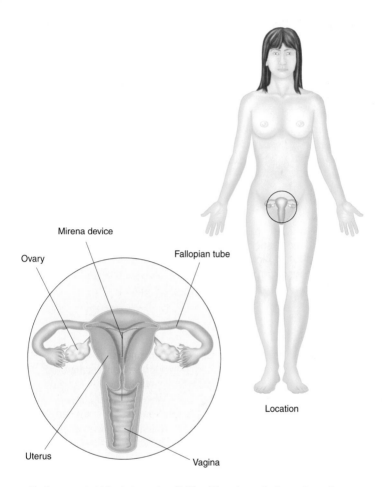

Location

The levonorgestrel intrauterine system (IUS) or Mirena is an effective contraceptive. It has a reservoir of progestogen that is slowly released directly into the uterus.

properties of oestrogen, progesterone and testosterone, in a single tablet. It is suitable for women whose periods have stopped because it is taken continuously. It relieves menopausal symptoms, while protecting the uterus and breast tissues from oestrogen stimulus. There is some evidence to suggest that tibolone is associated with a reduced risk of breast cancer compared with the standard oestrogen/progestogen HRT but further research is necessary to confirm these preliminary findings.

ADVANTAGES AND DISADVANTAGES OF DIFFERENT TYPES OF HRT

Advantages	Disadvantages
Tablets	
• Easy to take • Easily reversible • Cheap • Can combine with progestogen	• Unnatural delivery of hormone via the liver • Must be taken every day
Skin patches	
• Convenient • Easy to use • More natural delivery of hormone into the bloodstream • Easily reversible • Can combine with progestogen	• Can become detached • Can irritate the skin • More expensive than tablets • Must be changed once or twice a week
Gel	
• Easily reversible • Easy to use • More natural delivery of hormone into the bloodstream	• Must cover correct amount of skin • More expensive than tablets • Must use every day • If necessary, progestogen must be taken in a different formulation

Tibolone has the advantage of being period free. It can also be taken to prevent osteoporosis or to improve mood or libido. It is useful for women who are prone to breast tenderness with standard oestrogen therapy.

Unexpected bleeding is an occasional problem affecting around 10 to 15 per cent of users, and bleeding is more likely if the ovaries are still producing even small amounts of hormones. For this reason tibolone is recommended only for women who have not had a natural period for at least 12 months. This reduces the incidence of unnecessary investigations for erratic bleeding.

Advantages	Disadvantages
Nasal spray	
• Easy to use • More natural delivery of hormone into the bloodstream • Possibly fewer side effects than other routes • Easily reversible	• Nasal symptoms can be a problem but are usually mild • Long-term effects unknown • More expensive than tablets • Must use every day • If necessary, progestogen must be taken in a different formulation • Surges of oestrogen can aggravate conditions such as migraine
Implants	
• No missed doses • More natural delivery of hormones into the bloodstream • Prolonged effect: 4–12 months • Cheap	• Needs a small surgical procedure • Can cause unnaturally high levels of hormones • Not rapidly reversible • Progestogen must be continued for some time after the final implant
Vaginal	
• Useful if vaginal symptoms are the only problems • Easily reversible	• Some types of oestrogen are absorbed into the bloodstream • Progestogen may be necessary if used for longer than three months • Creams and pessaries can be messy

Raloxifene

Raloxifene (Evista) is the first of a new class of synthetic compounds known as selective oestrogen receptor modulators (SERMs). They mimic some of the actions of oestrogen but oppose others. Raloxifene has been shown to increase bone density in post-menopausal women, but not as effectively as oestrogen. It does not treat hot flushes or sweats, which may even occur as a side effect of use. Its theoretical advantage is that it does not stimulate the lining of the uterus. At present, it is recommended for the prevention of spinal fractures in postmenopausal women at risk of osteoporosis. Studies also suggest that raloxifene can reduce the risk of breast cancer, particularly oestrogen-dependent tumours. However, the risk of venous thrombosis is doubled in raloxifene users in the first years of use.

SAFETY ISSUES WITH OESTROGEN ± PROGESTERONE, TIBOLONE AND RALOXIFENE

	Oestrogen	Oestrogen + progestogen	Tibolone	Raloxifene
Breast	No change in risk	More risk	Possibly less risk	Possibly less risk
Endometrium (lining of uterus)	More risk	No change in risk	No change in risk	No change in risk
Heart disease and strokes	More risk	More risk	Less risk/no change in risk	More risk/no change in risk
Venous thrombosis	More risk	More risk	Less risk/no change in risk	More risk/no change in risk

EFFECTIVENESS OF OESTROGEN ± PROGESTERONE, TIBOLONE AND RALOXIFENE

	Oestrogen	Oestrogen + progestogen	Tibolone	Raloxifene
Bone density	Improves symptoms	Improves symptoms	Improves symptoms	Improves symptoms
Flushes and sweats	Improves symptoms	Improves symptoms	Improves symptoms	Symptoms may worsen
Vaginal symptoms	Improves symptoms	Improves symptoms	Improves symptoms	No change in symptoms

OESTROGEN–PROGESTOGEN COMBINATIONS

These sex hormone therapies combine oestrogen and progestogen and

Brand	Oestrogen	Dose
Climagest	Oestradiol valerate	1 or 2mg
Cyclo-Progynova	Oestradiol valerate	1 or 2mg
Elleste Duet	Oestradiol	1 or 2mg
Estracombi	Oestradiol	50µg
Evorel-Pak	Oestradiol	50µg
Evorel Sequi	Oestradiol	50µg
Femapak	Oestradiol	40 or 80µg
Femoston 1/10	Oestradiol	1mg
Femoston 2/10	Oestradiol	2mg
Femoston 2/20	Oestradiol	2mg
Femseven Sequi	Oestradiol	50µg
Femtab Sequi	Oestradiol	2mg
Novofem	Oestradiol	1mg
Nuvelle	Oestradiol valerate	2mg
Premique Cycle	Conjugated oestrogens	0.625mg
Prempak-C	Conjugated oestrogens	0.625 or 1.25mg
Tridestra	Oestradiol valerate	2mg

CONTINUOUS OESTROGEN–PROGESTOGEN

These preparations combine oestrogen and progestogen taken daily to

Brand	Oestrogen	Dose
Climesse	Oestradiol valerate	2mg
Elleste Duet Conti	Oestradiol	2mg
Evorel Conti	Oestradiol	50µg
Femoston Conti	Oestradiol	1mg
FemSeven Conti	Oestradiol	50µg
FemTab Continuous	Oestradiol	2mg
Indivina	Oestradiol	1 or 2mg
Kliofem	Oestradiol	2mg
Kliovance	Oestradiol	1mg
Nuvelle Continuous	Oestradiol hemihydrate	2mg
Premique Low Dose	Conjugated oestrogens	0.3mg
Premique	Conjugated oestrogens	0.625mg

produce a monthly or quarterly bleed.

Progestogen	Dose	Formulation	Bleed
Norethisterone	1 mg	Tablets	Monthly
Levonorgestrel	0.25 or 0.5 mg	Tablets	Monthly
Norethisterone	1 mg	Tablets	Monthly
Norethisterone	0.25 mg	Patches	Monthly
Norethisterone	1 mg	Patches/Tablets	Monthly
Norethisterone	170 µg	Patches	Monthly
Dydrogesterone	10 mg	Patches/Tablets	Monthly
Dydrogesterone	10 mg	Tablets	Monthly
Dydrogesterone	10 mg	Tablets	Monthly
Dydrogesterone	20 mg	Tablets	Monthly
Levonorgestrel	10 µg	Patches	Monthly
Levonorgestrel	75 µg	Tablets	Monthly
Norethisterone	1 mg	Tablets	Monthly
Levonorgestrel	75 µg	Tablets	Monthly
Medroxyprogesterone	10 mg	Tablets	Monthly
Norgestrel	150 µg	Tablets	Monthly
Medroxyprogesterone	20 mg	Tablets	Quarterly

avoid the need for a regular 'period'.

Progestogen	Dose	Formulation	Bleed
Norethisterone	0.7 mg	Tablets	No bleed
Norethisterone	1 mg	Tablets	No bleed
Norethisterone	170 µg	Patches	No bleed
Dydrogesterone	5 mg	Tablets	No bleed
Levonorgestrel	7 µg	Patches	No bleed
Norethisterone	1 mg	Tablets	No bleed
Medroxyprogesterone	2.5 or 5 mg	Tablets	No bleed
Norethisterone	1 mg	Tablets	No bleed
Norethisterone	0.5 mg	Tablets	No bleed
Norethisterone	1 mg	Tablets	No bleed
Medroxyprogesterone	1.5 mg	Tablets	No bleed
Medroxyprogesterone	5 mg	Tablets	No bleed

UNOPPOSED OESTROGEN

If you have had a hysterectomy only oestrogen treatment is necessary.

Brand	Oestrogen	Dose	Formulation
Aerodiol	Oestradiol hemihydrate	150 µg	Nasal spray
Climaval	Oestradiol	1 or 2 mg	Tablets
Elleste Solo	Oestradiol	1 or 2 mg	Tablets
Elleste Solo MX	Oestradiol	40 or 80 µg	Patches
Estraderm MX	Oestradiol	25, 50, 75 or 100 µg	Patches
Estraderm MX	Oestradiol	25, 50 or 100 µg	Patches
Evorel	Oestradiol	25, 50, 75 or 100 µg	Patches
Fematrix	Oestradiol	40 or 80 µg	Patches
FemSeven	Oestradiol	50, 75 or 100 µg	Patches
Femtab	Oestradiol valerate	1 or 2 mg	Tablets
Harmogen	Estropipate	1.5 mg	Tablets
Hormonin	Oestriol, oestrone and oestradiol		Tablets
Menoring	Oestradiol	50 µg	Vaginal ring
Oestrogel	Oestradiol	1.5 mg	Gel
Premarin	Conjugated oestrogens	0.625 or 1.25 mg	Tablets
Progynova	Oestradiol valerate	1 or 2 mg	Tablets
Progynova TS	Oestradiol	50 or 100 µg	Patches
Sandrena	Oestradiol	0.5 or 1 mg	Gel
Zumenon	Oestradiol	1 or 2 mg	Tablets

LOCAL OESTROGEN

Oestrogen can be applied directly (locally) to the area producing symptoms, for example, dry vagina. Use them strictly as prescribed because the oestrogen, if overused, can be absorbed through the skin into the bloodstream and affect the whole body.

Brand	Oestrogen	Dose	Formulation
Estring	Oestradiol	7.5 µg	Vaginal ring
Ortho-Gynest	Oestriol	0.5 mg	Vaginal pessary
Ortho-Gynest	Oestriol	0.01%	Vaginal cream
Ovestin	Oestriol	0.1%	Vaginal cream
Premarin	Conjugated oestrogens	0.0625%	Vaginal cream
Vagifem	Oestradiol	25 µg	Vaginal tablets

SELECTIVE TISSUE OESTROGENIC ACTIVITY REGULATOR (STEAR)

This preparation combines the properties of oestrogen, progestogen and testosterone.

Brand	Oestrogen	Dose	Formulation
Livial	Tibolone	2.5 mg	Tablets

SELECTIVE OESTROGEN RECEPTOR MODULATORS (SERMs)

SERMs mimic some of the actions of oestrogen. SERMs are used to treat postmenopausal osteoporosis.

Brand	Oestrogen	Dose	Formulation
Evista	Raloxifene	60 mg	Tablets

KEY POINTS

✓ There are different types of oestrogen and progestogen and some types may not suit you

✓ The hormones (oestrogen and progestogen) are taken cyclically during the climacteric but may be taken continuously once periods have stopped

✓ In addition to tablets, oestrogen is available as a patch, gel, nasal spray, vaginal ring or implant

✓ Each of these ways of taking hormones has different advantages and disadvantages

✓ Other more specific preparations are available, for example local oestrogen for vaginal dryness and testosterone for loss of interest in sex

How to take HRT

There are many different types of HRT. For women who have had a hysterectomy, most need take only oestrogen, otherwise they need to take progestogen as well to protect them from cancer of the lining of the uterus. Sometimes women who have had a hysterectomy because of endometriosis are advised to take additional progestogens. Endometriosis occurs when the endometrium, the lining of the uterus, is found outside the uterus in other parts of the body. It is stimulated by oestrogen and suppressed by progestogen – hence the benefits of the latter hormone.

WOMEN WITH A UTERUS
Sequential combined HRT
This is oestrogen combined with cyclical progestogen and is the HRT that most women use. Oestrogen is taken continuously, without a break. It can be taken daily as a tablet, once or twice a week as a patch, or as a gel, nasal spray, vaginal ring or implant. Progestogen is added every month, either as a course of tablets lasting 10 to 14 days or as a combined patch with oestrogen, replaced twice weekly.

Calendar packs are available to help remember when to take the progestogen. If oestrogen and progestogen are prescribed separately, most doctors recommend that the progestogen course is started on the first day of every calendar month. All these forms of HRT should give a withdrawal bleed around or shortly after the end of the progestogen course. Any unexpected bleeding should be reported to the doctor.

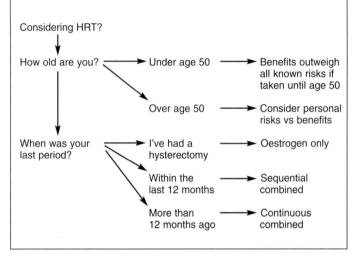

IS HRT RIGHT FOR YOU?

You may find this flowchart useful to help with your choices.

Considering HRT?

How old are you? → Under age 50 → Benefits outweigh all known risks if taken until age 50

Over age 50 → Consider personal risks vs benefits

When was your last period? → I've had a hysterectomy → Oestrogen only

Within the last 12 months → Sequential combined

More than 12 months ago → Continuous combined

More recently, long-cycle HRT has been introduced. This involves taking oestrogen every day as usual, but taking the progestogen course only every three months. This means that there are only four withdrawal bleeds every year. A disadvantage of this regimen is that a relatively high dose of progestogen is needed, which can give side effects such as bloating, headaches and irritability, as well as heavy and/or prolonged bleeding. Despite this, long-cycle HRT is useful for women whose natural periods are infrequent.

Sequential combined HRT

Oestrogen daily

Progestogen

Period

Month 1   Month 2   Month 3   Month 4

Long-cycle combined HRT

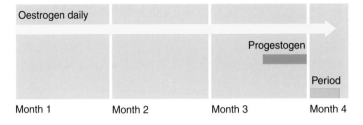

Oestrogen daily			
		Progestogen	
			Period
Month 1	Month 2	Month 3	Month 4

Continuous combined HRT

Most women who have gone through the menopause do not wish to return to monthly periods. To avoid this, a combination of oestrogen and progestogen is taken daily. Taking both hormones together prevents any thickening of the uterine lining, making a withdrawal bleed unnecessary while providing protection against endometrial cancer. Although it can be taken by premenopausal women, irregular bleeding is a common problem.

Even in postmenopausal women, unpredictable bleeding may occur during the first few months, sometimes heavy and prolonged. However, in most woman who persevere, bleeding usually settles within 12 months. Bleeding is less likely the longer the woman has been postmenopausal before starting the treatment. So continuous combined HRT is generally recommended only if the woman has been postmenopausal for at least a year. In such cases,

continuous combined HRT can be highly satisfactory, although missed pills can often lead to some spotting.

If you are postmenopausal and have been taking cyclical HRT but want to change to a period-free type, you should start your new tablets at the end of a withdrawal bleed, which is usually several days into a fresh pack of your old cyclical HRT. This reduces the likelihood of any unwanted bleeding, because your uterine lining is already thin when you start your new HRT.

A recent advance has been to give continuous oestrogen to women who are using the progestogen-releasing intrauterine system, IUS (Mirena), used for contraception. This has a particular advantage for women who are at risk of pregnancy. It also keeps the uterine lining thin because the progestogen is released directly into the uterus and has few side effects. The IUS is also used to relieve painful or heavy periods. Although it is widely used together

Continuous combined HRT

| Month 1 | Month 2 | Month 3 | Month 4 |

Oestrogen daily

Progestogen daily

with oestrogen for HRT, it is not currently licensed (see Glossary on page 111) for this indication in the UK. As with other period-free regimens, irregular bleeding can occur in the first few months but this usually settles quickly.

Cyclical oestrogen

Oestrogen treatment used to be given for three out of every four weeks, with no progestogen therapy. But with this treatment, menopausal symptoms returned during the oestrogen-free week and the risk of endometrial cancer is increased. It is no longer recommended in the UK, but is still prescribed in some other countries. Those women who take oestrogen in this way should see a doctor and discuss other forms of HRT.

WOMEN WHO HAVE HAD A HYSTERECTOMY

Continuous oestrogen

Women who have had a hysterectomy have the advantage of not needing to take progestogen. This reduces the likelihood of unwanted side effects. They can take daily oestrogen tablets, once- or twice-weekly patches, daily gel, daily nasal spray, a three-monthly vaginal ring or six-monthly implants.

WOMEN WHO HAVE VAGINAL SYMPTOMS ONLY

Local oestrogen

Topical oestrogen delivered directly into the vagina is very useful for local symptoms in the absence of other menopausal symptoms. They are available as creams, pessaries, tablets and a vaginal ring. Symptoms usually respond within three months of starting treatment but it can take up to a year of continuous use before a benefit is noticed. Most brands of vaginal oestrogen result in very little absorption into the bloodstream so, if used short term (up to three months), no additional progestogen therapy is necessary. However, if conjugated equine oestrogen cream is used, or if other local oestrogen is used long term, additional progestogen may be necessary, unless the woman has had a hysterectomy. If she is using vaginal oestrogen and experiences unexpected bleeding, she must see her doctor.

WHAT IS THE RIGHT DOSE OF HRT?

How much oestrogen?

The dose of oestrogen taken depends on the reason why it is being taken. Relief of severe symptoms requires a higher dose than relief of mild symptoms. Younger women also need higher doses to get the same benefit as older women. Many women wonder why their hormone levels are not tested – this is because normal oestrogen levels vary so much that it is more appropriate to monitor symptom control. If symptoms are not adequately controlled, the dose of oestrogen needs increasing; if side effects are a problem, the dose is too high. Research suggests that even low doses can protect against osteoporosis.

How much progestogen?

The dose of progestogen has to be high enough to eliminate the risk of cancer of the lining of the uterus (endometrial cancer) almost completely. However, unnecessarily high doses should be avoided because progestogen may increase the risk of breast cancer when taken with oestrogen.

KEY POINTS

✓ Unless a woman has had a hysterectomy, she must use progestogen in addition to oestrogen, in order to protect her uterine lining from cancer

✓ Women going through the menopause usually use sequential combined HRT, with a withdrawal bleed when they stop the progestogen each month

✓ Postmenopausal women can use continuous combined HRT and do not have to have periods

✓ The lowest dose of oestrogen necessary to treat menopausal symptoms is recommended

HRT: when to start and when to stop

WHEN SHOULD YOU START HRT?

The best time to start HRT depends on your personal circumstances, the likely balance of risks versus benefits and your personal preference. HRT is usually started around the menopause in order to control hot flushes and sweats. However, it can be started at any age, if there is good reason to do so.

HOW LONG SHOULD YOU TAKE HRT FOR?

Most women take HRT for a couple of years, in order to treat menopausal symptoms. If taken for up to five years, there is no evidence that it increases the risk of breast cancer. Some women continue to have severe menopausal symptoms

beyond five years. For these women HRT remains an effective option, particularly if non-hormonal treatments are not effective.

However, long-term use can be associated with increased risk of breast cancer and this is higher with combined HRT than with oestrogen-only HRT. There is also an increased risk of venous thrombosis and stroke. Most of these risks increase with increasing age anyway, not just with HRT use. Only you can decide whether the benefits of HRT outweigh these potential risks. Your decision will depend on how troublesome your menopausal symptoms are to you.

Women in their 60s or older who need treatment to prevent osteoporosis are usually advised to consider non-hormonal treatments first. Some women prefer to choose HRT. However, in order to prevent osteoporosis, life-long treatment is necessary because bone loss begins as soon as HRT is stopped.

Some women wish to continue HRT lifelong, just because it makes them feel so well. There is no reason why they should not do this, provided that the benefit is carefully weighed against the risk.

Women who have had a premature menopause, either spontaneously or through surgical removal of the ovaries, are at no additional risk from HRT use when taken until they are 50, no matter for how many years they take it. This is because HRT is replacing the hormones that would normally be produced until the natural menopause.

How do you stop HRT?

HRT maintains a hormonal balance, levelling out the hormonal fluctuations that are responsible for menopausal symptoms. Stopping HRT suddenly will provoke an abrupt drop in oestrogen and symptoms return. When this happens, the symptoms result from the sudden change in HRT and do not necessarily reflect what is happening with your own hormones.

To avoid this, and to enable you to assess whether or not menopausal symptoms caused by your own hormones have abated, you should gradually reduce the oestrogen dose over a period of two to six months, typically by cutting pills or matrix patches (patches will not leak if cut) into increasingly smaller doses or using increasingly smaller amounts of gel. This allows the level to decline gradually, minimising the likelihood of symptoms developing. You must continue to take the same progestogen dose, in the usual way, until you have completely stopped the oestrogen.

Women using oestrogen implants can also gradually reduce the dose of each implant when it is replaced every six months. However, the effects of an implant on the uterine lining can continue for up to two to three years. So, unless the woman has had a hysterectomy, she must continue taking progestogen until the implant has worn off. This can be assessed by whether or not a withdrawal bleed occurs following a course of progestogen. If it does, then oestrogen is still present, causing the lining of the uterus to thicken. If there is no bleeding, it is usually safe to stop taking progestogen.

KEY POINTS

✓ HRT can be started at any age but is most often started around the menopause to control flushes and sweats

✓ If taken for up to five years beyond the menopause, there are no major risks

✓ HRT can be taken lifelong but using it for more than five years carries increased risks

✓ Women who have a premature menopause should take HRT until they are 50; this is not associated with any increased risks because it is replacing hormones that would have normally been present

✓ Suddenly stopping HRT can result in the return of flushes and sweats resulting from a sudden drop in oestrogen – this can be minimised by reducing the oestrogen dose over several months

Side effects of HRT

Around 35 per cent of women stop taking HRT because of unwanted side effects. Often, these side effects could be resolved by a change in the dose or type of HRT. So it is very important to discuss feelings and experiences with the doctor before just stopping HRT. If a women decides to stop, she should talk to her doctor about how best to do this (see previous chapter).

Side effects of oestrogen

Fluid retention, bloating, breast tenderness, nausea, leg cramps and gastric upset are symptoms associated with high levels of oestrogen, and are not uncommon when starting HRT. If they have not settled by the end of the third month from starting HRT, it is worth considering lowering your oestrogen dose or changing to a different form of HRT.

Leg cramps can improve with exercise and regular stretching of the calf muscles. Gastric upsets usually improve if oral HRT is taken with food. Breast tenderness is sometimes alleviated by a low-fat, low-carbohydrate diet. Evening primrose oil can also help.

Side effects of progestogen

Side effects are much more common with cyclical courses than with continuous progestogen. The most

SIDE EFFECTS OF OESTROGEN AND PROGESTOGEN

Oestrogen and progestogen are associated with a number of side effects. Some of the most frequently occurring side effects that women may experience when they start HRT are listed below. Many resolve within the first two to three months.

Oestrogen	Progestogen
Fluid retention	Fluid retention
Feeling of bloatedness	Breast tenderness
Breast tenderness	Depression
Nausea	Nausea
Stomach upset	Irritability
Leg cramps	Headaches
	Mood swings
	Abdominal pain
	Backache
	Acne

common problem is 'premenstrual' symptoms, which affect up to 20 per cent of women taking cyclical progestogen. These symptoms include fluid retention, breast tenderness, mood swings, depression, acne, lower abdominal pains and backache. They are most apparent when starting HRT and often resolve with continued use.

If they persist, altering the dose or type of progestogen can help. Changing the route of delivery can also help – for example, from tablets to patches.

If symptoms are particularly severe, the progestogen course could be taken every three months rather than monthly. Alternatively, the duration of the progestogen could be shortened, but reducing the course to less than ten days reduces the protective effect against cancer of the lining of the uterus and can provoke irregular bleeding.

Postmenopausal women can change to continuous combined HRT, which requires a lower dose of progestogen than cyclical regimens and has the advantage of being period free.

OTHER EFFECTS OF HRT

Bleeding

Unless you have had a hyster-ectomy, you will probably need cyclical progestogen, taken as a course, usually as tablets or patches, every month. If you are taking cyclical progestogen, a withdrawal bleed or 'period' usually starts around the end of the progestogen course.

It is useful to keep a record of when you use the progestogen and when your period starts. If your bleeding starts early in the pro-gestogen course or if you get bleeding unexpectedly at other times of the month, you should report this to your doctor. It is quite common in the first few months of taking HRT, but if unusual bleeding starts after taking HRT for six months or longer, the cause needs to be assessed.

You may only need to change the dose, timing, duration or type of progestogen but your doctor may want to check that the progestogen is providing adequate protection against cancerous changes develop-ing in the uterus.

In many gynaecology depart-ments, one of the first steps after a manual internal examination has been done is to arrange for you to have a transvaginal (TVS) ultrasound scan. A small probe is inserted into the vagina and the ultrasound waves create a picture of the uterus and ovaries. A TVS can also be used to measure the thickness of the endometrium and identify common benign causes of bleeding such as fibroids or polyps.

Transducer

Ultrasound screen

During a transvaginal ultrasound scan (TVS) a small probe is inserted into the vagina and the ultrasound waves create a picture of the uterus and ovaries.

Some doctors perform an endometrial biopsy. This involves taking a small sample of the lining of the uterus. It can be done in the outpatient department, without the need for an anaesthetic, and you can go home immediately after. A thin hollow rod is inserted through your cervix, into the uterus. A small sample of tissue is then scraped from the endometrial lining of the uterus. You may feel some

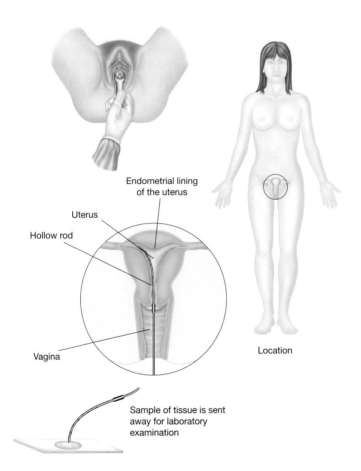

Endometrial lining of the uterus

Uterus

Hollow rod

Vagina

Location

Sample of tissue is sent away for laboratory examination

During an endometrial biopsy a small sample is taken from the lining of the uterus.

cramping pains but these usually pass very quickly. It is usual for some spotting to occur for a few hours after.

Most hospitals can now perform a hysteroscopy in the outpatient department. Although this investigation has the advantage of enabling the doctor to look directly at the endometrium, it is a longer procedure than a TVS or endometrial biopsy. A long thin rod with a video camera and a light attached to it is inserted into the uterus. The uterus is distended slightly by pumping in carbon dioxide gas or saline (salt water), allowing the doctor to look at the endometrium. Small scissors can be inserted through the rod to take samples. By using local anaesthesia, there is usually minimal discomfort during hysteroscopy. If someone is very anxious, it is possible to give a short-acting narcotic intravenously. Most women are able to get up and return to their normal activities immediately, although mild cramps

Uterus is distended with carbon dioxide or salt water

Uterus

Vagina

Viewing screen

Hysteroscope

Location

A hysteroscopy has the advantage of enabling the doctor to look inside the uterus, and samples of the endometrial tissue can also be taken.

INVESTIGATING SUSPICIOUS BLEEDING

Unexpected bleeding may be an indication of an underlying problem needing specific treatment and is usually investigated by one of the following techniques.

Technique	Anaesthetic required?
Endometrial biopsy: taking a sample of the lining of the uterus using a narrow hollow rod	No
Transvaginal ultrasound scan (TVS): a small probe is inserted into the vagina to view the uterus and ovaries	No
Hysteroscopy: a camera is inserted into the uterus to look at the endometrium and enable direct samples of the tissue to be taken	Sometimes

and some bloody discharge may occur for a day or two.

WEIGHT GAIN

Although many women are concerned that HRT will make them put on weight, studies show that HRT users often gain less weight than non-users after the menopause. A few women are sensitive to oral oestrogen, particularly if the dose is too high, causing them to retain fluid and gain weight. Simply reducing the dose or changing to a non-oral form can resolve this.

HEADACHES

Fluctuating hormone levels can trigger migraine and headaches. These fluctuations are common with oral forms of HRT (taken by mouth). Switching to a non-oral form may solve the problem.

KEY POINTS

✓ Side effects are common when starting HRT but most resolve in the first two to three months

✓ If side effects persist, they must be discussed with a doctor because there are various ways to minimise them

✓ Often side effects can be resolved by a change in dose or type of HRT

✓ One way is to try a lower dose of progestogen but it must be enough to protect from endometrial cancer

✓ A different route of delivery may relieve side effects – for example, change from tablets to patches

HRT: who can and who can't take it

There are very few conditions that prevent women from using HRT. However, there is often some misinformation about who can and who can't take it.

WHO CAN TAKE HRT?

Women with any of the following conditions can use HRT, although some may need specialist supervision:

- Cervical cancer
- Coeliac (non-oral route preferred)
- Crohn's disease (non-oral route preferred)
- Diabetes
- Epilepsy
- High blood pressure (non-oral route preferred)
- High cholesterol (route depends on lipid profile)
- Kidney failure
- Mild liver disease (non-oral route preferred)
- Malignant melanoma
- Migraine (non-oral route preferred)
- Ovarian cancer
- Parkinson's disease
- Rheumatoid arthritis
- Thyroid disease
- Heart valve disease.

WHO SHOULD BE CAUTIOUS ABOUT HRT?

Benign breast lumps

There is no convincing evidence that this condition is associated with a greater than expected risk of breast cancer in women using HRT.

If a woman has breast lumps, they should be checked before starting HRT to make sure that they are not cancerous. Regular checks should be continued once treatment has begun.

Endometriosis

Sometimes the tissue that lines the uterus is found in abnormal sites such as the rectum or navel. In the same way that the lining of the uterus is shed each month during menstruation, these other sites also bleed, causing severe pain and heavy periods. This condition, known as endometriosis, is stimulated by oestrogen and improves with the menopause.

HRT can occasionally reactivate the condition so if you have had endometriosis you should be cautious when taking HRT, monitoring any symptoms particularly of pain on intercourse and heavy or irregular bleeding. Even if you have had a hysterectomy, some doctors will recommend that you take continuous progestogen to prevent the endometriosis recurring. This is because the lining of the uterus cannot grow in the presence of progestogen.

Fibroids

Fibroids (non-cancerous growths in the muscle of the uterus) are very common. They are sensitive to oestrogen so they often grow during pregnancy as the level of oestrogen in the body rises, and shrink after the menopause. As a result of this, fibroids can enlarge with HRT, causing heavy withdrawal bleeding. Continuous progestogen can reduce the likelihood of fibroids increasing in size. The levonorgestrel intrauterine system (see pages 63–64) is sometimes used to help treat fibroids.

Gallstones

If you have gallstones you should discuss HRT use with your doctor because the gallstones may enlarge, particularly with oral therapy. If you have had problems with gallstones in the past, some doctors suggest that you should use patches or implants rather than tablets to reduce the amount of oestrogen passing through the liver. It is safe to use HRT if you have had an operation to remove gallstones.

Otosclerosis

Otosclerosis is an inherited cause of hearing loss caused by the growth of extra bone which prevents the small bones in the ear from working properly. This condition can deteriorate rapidly during pregnancy, suggesting a link with oestrogen. HRT may have the same effect, so specialist advice should be sought before starting treatment.

WHO SHOULD NOT TAKE HRT?

Breast cancer

There are two main types of breast cancers – those that are sensitive to oestrogen and those that are not. If you have been successfully treated for non-oestrogen-dependent breast cancer you may still be able to take HRT, particularly if you have a specific reason to do so – such as relieving severe hot flushes. However, you need to be carefully supervised by a specialist. Even women with oestrogen-dependent cancers can usually take vaginal oestrogen to treat local symptoms.

Endometrial cancer

The majority of women found to have endometrial cancer are likely to be cured by hysterectomy. Following successful surgery, many women subsequently develop debilitating menopausal symptoms, which may not always respond to non-hormonal treatment. If a woman with a history of endometrial cancer develops symptoms that warrant HRT, it can usually be prescribed. However, because endometrial cancer is oestrogen dependent, most doctors prescribe progestogen as well as oestrogen in order to minimise the likelihood of recurrence.

Severe liver disease

You should not take HRT if you have jaundice as a result of severe liver disease. This is because most of the oestrogen, particularly if taken by mouth, is broken down by your liver, increasing its metabolic load. This is not a problem for a healthy liver but a diseased liver may not be able to cope with this extra workload. If your jaundice improves and your liver works normally again, then there is no reason why HRT should not be taken. Non-oral forms – patches or implants – are recommended because lower hormone levels pass through the liver.

Blood clots (venous thrombosis)

Venous thrombosis can result from an underlying genetic condition or a blood clotting disorder (thrombophilia). If you have a close family member who had an unexplained blood clot under the age of 45, investigations to screen for thrombophilia or underlying disease may be necessary before HRT can be considered.

Heart attacks and strokes

It is not recommended that you should start HRT in order to try to prevent heart attacks or strokes if you have already experienced one. However, if you have a history of either of these, you may be given HRT if you have severe menopausal symptoms or are at risk of osteoporosis. If you have had a heart attack or stroke and are already taking HRT, this is not a reason to stop it.

Pregnancy

Despite fertility being low as women approach the menopause, it is still possible to become pregnant. Most HRTs are not contraceptive. Women who have taken HRT and then found that they are pregnant can be reassured that it is unlikely that HRT will adversely affect outcome of pregnancy. However, miscarriage rates are high in older women for other reasons.

Undiagnosed vaginal bleeding

HRT should not be used to control unusual bleeding until the cause of the bleeding has been assessed. This is because HRT itself can cause unexpected bleeding and mask an underlying problem that may need treatment.

KEY POINTS

✓ Few women are unable to take HRT on medical grounds

✓ HRT is not recommended if you have oestrogen-dependent cancers such as cancer of the endometrium or oestrogen-dependent breast cancer

✓ You should not start HRT while you have venous thrombosis, active liver disease or unexplained vaginal bleeding

Controlling symptoms without HRT

Although HRT is the 'gold standard' for controlling menopausal symptoms, relieving up to 80 per cent of hot flushes, not every woman can, needs to or wants to take it. For many women, particularly those with mild symptoms, one or other of the following options can be effective.

CONTROLLING HOT FLUSHES

Many women use non-prescription remedies to treat hot flushes, such as isoflavones. Also popular are dong quai, evening primrose oil, vitamin E, ginseng, liquorice and natural progesterone creams. Most of these are classed as dietary supplements and so are not regulated in the same way as drugs. Hence these treatments can be sold in health shops, supermarkets and pharmacies without evidence that they are either effective or safe. Also, information about how they interact with other therapies and prescription drugs is often limited.

Isoflavones

These plant oestrogens are often called phytoestrogens. Two common sources of isoflavones are soy and red clover. The recommended dose is 40 to 80 mg a day – the same dose used in most of the studies using isoflavones for the treatment of hot flushes, but it can

take several weeks before any benefit is seen. The potential for toxic or
adverse side effects with these doses
is minimal. Soy products or foods
fortified with soy are often advertised
as alleviating flushes but supplements allow a consistent daily intake.

Black cohosh

Preparations made from the thick
underground stems (rhizomes) of
the herb black cohosh have been
studied, with varying reports of
efficacy. Almost all the studies have
used different formulations and
doses, so the results are difficult to
compare. Although a popular
remedy, black cohosh is not recommended because there have been
reports of toxic effects on the liver
with long-term use.

Dong quai

This herb is commonly used in
traditional Chinese medicine to treat
gynaecological problems. Studies
using the herb to control hot flushes
have shown little benefit. Women
using warfarin should not take dong
quai.

Evening primrose oil

Although very effective for treating
breast tenderness premenstrually,
even high doses of evening primrose oil (two grams daily) have
shown little benefit for hot flushes.
Side effects include nausea and
diarrhoea.

Vitamin E

Studies using vitamin E in doses up
to 400 IU twice daily have not
shown much effect on hot flushes.
Side effects are few and not serious.

Ginseng

Studies with ginseng have not
shown benefit on hot flushes.
Ginseng can adversely interact with
monoamine oxidase inhibitors
(MAOIs), which may be prescribed
for treatment of depression, and
with anticoagulants such as aspirin
and warfarin.

Liquorice

The root of the liquorice plant is
used in many Chinese preparations
for menopausal symptoms. However,
there are no studies to show either
safety or efficacy. Women taking
diuretics should not use liquorice.
High doses of liquorice can cause
fluid retention and high blood
pressure.

Natural progesterone cream

Progesterone is synthesised by a
chemical process from plants such
as soy beans or wild yam. Some of
the products contain progesterone
indistinguishable from a woman's
own natural progesterone. Others
contain only chemical precursors of
progesterone found in plants, which
are inactive in humans because
they cannot be converted to progesterone. As these creams are

regulated as dietary supplements, it is not possible to know which products are which.

Although creams containing progesterone, often combined with vitamin E and aloe vera, have shown a positive effect on flushes there are safety concerns about unregulated hormonal treatments. Women using oestrogen replacement therapy should not use progesterone creams in place of prescribed progestogens (synthetic progesterones), because they may not protect the endometrium.

REDUCING HOT FLUSHES WITHOUT HORMONAL TREATMENT

Some women prefer to try non-prescription and non-hormonal remedies to control hot flushes. These include herbal and homoeopathic options. If these do not work, women should ask their GPs to consider which of the non-hormonal prescriptions (in other words not HRT) are suitable for them.

Serotonin inhibitors

Serotonin is a neurotransmitter in the brain and is important in the control of mood and behaviour, feeding and hunger, temperature regulation and sleep. Selective serotonin reuptake inhibitors (SSRIs) are licensed for the treatment of depression. Depression is caused by low serotonin levels and SSRIs increase the serotonin levels. However, research has also shown that lower doses of SSRIs are effective for a wide variety of other conditions, including control of chronic pain conditions, migraine and hot flushes. The three most commonly used for hot flushes are venlafaxine (Efexor), paroxetine (Seroxat) and fluoxetine (Prozac). Trials suggest that there can be up to a 60 per cent reduction in flushes. Although symptoms can improve immediately, it may take up to eight weeks before any benefit is seen. The most common side effects are nausea, weight loss and reduced sex drive.

Gabapentin

This drug is licensed for the control of epilepsy but is also used for chronic pain conditions. and can halve the rate of hot flushes. Side effects include dizziness and feeling light-headed as well as some fluid retention and tiredness. As antacids (indigestion remedies) can reduce the amount of gabapentin that gets into the body, gabapentin should be taken at least two hours after an antacid is used.

Clonidine

This drug, originally developed for the treatment of high blood pressure, can alleviate mild hot flushes but is less effective than SSRIs or gabapentin. Side effects of drowsiness, dizziness, constipation and depression are common.

OTHER NON-HRT TREATMENTS

Combined oral contraceptives (see pages 99–100)

Combined oral contraceptives (COCs), containing synthetic oestrogen (ethinyloestradiol) and synthetic progesterone (progestogen), inhibit ovulation. Healthy, non-smoking women can take low-dose COCs right up to the menopause. They provide contraception and prevent hot flushes but the doses of hormones are much higher than HRT. This means that the risk of blood clots is greater than for HRT but benefits, particularly of lighter menstrual periods, can make COCs a good option for some women.

Progestogen

Although progestogen is usually taken together with oestrogen for HRT, high-dose progestogen can be effective on its own. Medroxy-progesterone acetate or MPA (Depo-Provera) can be given by injection every three months and also provides contraception. The side effects can include weight gain and irregular bleeding. There is also some controversy about the effect of injectable MPA on bone density. MPA tablets, 20 mg a day, are also effective and result in less irregular bleeding. It can take up to six weeks to reach its maximum effect. Another progestogen tablet, megestrol acetate, 20 mg twice a day, is also effective.

KEY POINTS

✓ HRT is the most effective treatment for menopausal symptoms

✓ Non-hormonal remedies such as dietary isoflavones may alleviate mild symptoms in some women

✓ For more severe symptoms, venlafaxine, paroxetine, fluoxetine or gabapentin is available on prescription

Contraception around the menopause

Women approaching the menopause often wrongly assume that they no longer need to use contraception. It is certainly true that a woman in her 40s is about half as fertile as a woman in her 20s. Also, her eggs are of a poorer quality and ovulation is less regular, until she finally stops ovulating and experiences the menopause. Despite this, pregnancy can occur. If you are not protected and your periods suddenly stop, you might assume it is the menopause, but it could be that you are pregnant.

Although many babies born to older mothers are very healthy, genetic abnormalities such as Down's syndrome become more common. The risk of miscarriage and risks to mother and baby are also increased in older women.

Therefore effective contraception can be as important for a woman in her late 40s as it is for a woman in her teens or 20s.

Contraception should be continued for at least 12 months after the last period in women over the age of 50. Women who have an earlier menopause are advised to continue contraception for at least two years after the last period.

HORMONAL CONTRACEPTION

Combined hormonal contraceptives

Combined oral contraceptives (COCs; commonly known as the pill), the contraceptive patch and the contraceptive vaginal ring, contain both synthetic oestrogen and progestogen. They work by inhibiting ovulation. In addition to their contraceptive effects, they will also provide relief from menopausal symptoms. Healthy, non-smoking women can use modern, low-dose, combined hormonal contraceptives until one or two years after the menopause. Although synthetic oestrogens increase the risk of blood clots, this has to be balanced against potential health benefits for perimenopausal women including relief of premenstrual symptoms and regular periods that are less painful and heavy than natural periods. There is also some evidence that combined oral contraceptives have a positive effect on bone density.

Progestogen-only methods

Although postmenopausal use of progestogen is associated with increased risk of breast cancer, there is no evidence of this effect when progestogens are taken before the menopause. The advantage of progestogen-only methods over combined hormonal contraception is that there is no associated increased risk of blood clots with the former. There are several types of contraception that contain just progestogen. Each of them works in a slightly different way. Progestogen-only methods can be prescribed to many women at risk of blood clots who cannot use combined hormonal contraceptives, including smokers.

- **Progestogen-only pill**: The progestogen-only pill (POP), also known as the mini-pill, is taken every day and contains a very low dose of progestogen. Unlike COCs, which inhibit ovulation, standard POPs have minimal effect on ovulation but act by thickening cervical mucus and preventing sperm getting into the uterus. For women over 35, standard POPs are as effective as combined oral contraceptives. A newer POP, called Cerazette, does inhibit ovulation. The main potential problem with POPs is irregular bleeding. This may be resolved by changing to a different type of POP. In contrast, some women find that their periods stop.

- **Injectables**: There are two types of progestogen that can be injected: depot medroxyprogesterone acetate (DMPA; Depo-Provera) and norethisterone acetate (NETA; Noristerat). As with the combined pill, they work by inhibiting the monthly release of the egg from the ovaries. Both types are administered by health-care professionals by deep intramuscular injection into the buttock or upper arm: DMPA every twelve weeks and NETA every eight weeks. Injectables can relieve premenstrual symptoms and heavy, painful periods. They can be associated with weight gain and irregular bleeding, although this usually resolves with continued use.

- **Implant:** Implanon is a single rod, about the size of a hairgrip, which contains progestogen. It works by switching off the normal menstrual cycle, similar to the combined pill and injectables. A trained health-care professional injects the rod just under the skin on the inner side of the upper arm. It is both palpable and visible after insertion but is a highly effective contraceptive, lasting for up to three years.

It is not licensed (see Glossary, page 111) for use in women aged over 40, although you can use it if you and your doctor think it is a suitable method for you. Implants can relieve many period-related problems, particularly heavy, painful periods. The main drawbacks can be weight gain and irregular bleeding, which can be frequent or prolonged in up to 20 per cent of users.

Levonorgestrel intrauterine system

The levonorgestrel intrauterine system (Mirena) is a small T-shaped device containing progestogen inserted into the uterus by trained health-care professionals. Progestogen is released directly into the uterus, keeping the uterine lining or endometrium thin (important for lower risk of endometrial cancer). Side effects are few as the hormonal effect is essentially within the uterus, and only small amounts of hormone reach the bloodstream. The IUS is as effective as sterilisation but is easily reversed by removal of the device. It is also an effective treatment for heavy, painful periods. In addition to its use as a contraceptive, the IUS can also be used together with natural oestrogen supplements as HRT. Occasionally, irregular, frequent or prolonged bleeding can necessitate removal of the device.

NON-HORMONAL CONTRACEPTION

Sterilisation

Both vasectomy and female sterilisation are popular in older couples. However, sterilisation needs to be considered very carefully because this method is essentially irreversible. Many reversible methods such as the IUS and implants are as effective as sterilisation, often with added benefits for period-related problems.

Copper intrauterine device

Modern intrauterine devices (IUDs), often called coils, offer highly effective reversible contraception. They contain copper, which kills sperm before they can reach the uterus. If inserted after your fortieth birthday, an IUD can remain in place until after your menopause. The main disadvantage of this method is increased menstrual blood loss and period pains, so it is not recommended if you already have heavy or painful periods.

Barrier methods

Barrier methods can be sufficiently effective in older women because their fertility is lower. Condoms (including the female condom Femidom) are the most popular barrier method and are widely available without prescription. Polyurethane condoms are available for those with latex allergy. Diaphragms are popular with many couples and new female barrier methods are now available over the counter.

Vaginal sponge

A small, one-size, single-use disposable vaginal sponge is available over the counter. It is impregnated with three different spermicides. In addition to the effects of the spermicides, the sponge forms a physical barrier over the cervix and absorbs sperm.

Spermicides

In women over age 50, a spermicide can be sufficient on its own because fertility is so low. It can also help vaginal lubrication.

Coitus interruptus

Coitus interruptus or the withdrawal method is not a reliable contraceptive at any age and you should consider other more effective methods.

Fertility awareness

Methods such as measuring changes in temperature, checking cervical secretions and calculating the 'safe period' can be very effective for motivated women with regular menstrual periods. These methods become less reliable during the menopause as periods become erratic.

WHEN CAN YOU STOP USING CONTRACEPTION?

If you are over 50, contraception can be stopped one year after your periods end. If you are under 50 and your periods stop, you should continue using contraception for another two years after what you believe to be the last period, provided that your periods do not return in that time. Barrier methods, spermicides alone or the contraceptive sponge is sufficient at these times because your fertility is low.

As most women's natural periods stop around the age of 50, it is generally advisable to stop hormonal contraception when you are about that age and change to alternative contraception until you know that you are past the menopause.

HRT AND CONTRACEPTION

HRT does not restore fertility, nor is it always an effective contraceptive. Therefore, if you start HRT before your periods have stopped naturally, there is a risk of pregnancy.

Most standard HRT methods are not contraceptive so additional non-hormonal contraception is usually recommended. One HRT regime increasingly recommended is to use the progestogen-containing contraceptive IUS (Mirena) in conjunction with oestrogen.

Withdrawal bleeds associated with some types of HRT can make it difficult to assess the timing of your natural menopause. Blood tests (see pages 7–8) can be taken in the oestrogen-only phase of the sequential combined HRT and may sometimes indicate the menopause, but it is usually necessary to stop HRT to achieve a valid result. Otherwise contraception should be continued until you are 55 when it is safe to assume that you are no longer fertile.

KEY POINTS

✓ Contraception is important if you are at risk of becoming pregnant

✓ Most standard methods of HRT are not contraceptive so additional non-hormonal contraception may be necessary

✓ Some hormonal methods of contraception also provide HRT

✓ Contraception can be stopped two years after your last natural period if you are under 50, and one year after your last natural period if you are over 50

✓ If you don't want to stop HRT to find out if you have gone through the menopause you should continue contraception until you are 55

HRT: conclusions

HRT has been available to women for over 60 years but for much of that time guidance for prescription has been based on biased observational studies. This has led to the false belief that HRT is a panacea for all age-related ailments in women.

Now we are fortunate to have the results from well-designed studies comparing HRT with inactive treatment, enabling us to assess more accurately the true benefits and risks of HRT. From these studies we see that certain types of HRT, notably conjugated oral oestrogens taken together with the progestogen medroxyprogesterone acetate, when given to post-menopausal women, can increase the risk of stroke, heart disease, venous thrombosis and breast cancer. In contrast, oestrogen-only HRT does not appear to increase the risk of breast cancer and all studies confirm the benefits of HRT on treating menopause symptoms, reducing the risk of fractures of the hip and spine and of colorectal cancer.

On the basis of these results, recent recommendations for HRT have been amended to ensure that women are most likely to benefit from the prescription with minimal risks. Hence HRT remains an effective treatment for menopause symptoms but is no longer recommended to prevent stroke.

Current recommendations correctly endorse that HRT should be prescribed on an individual basis and for the shortest time necessary. This is not defined by an arbitrary time limit but depends on the individual needs of the woman, who is fully informed about the pros and cons of HRT.

Although guidelines based on accurate evidence are laudable, it is important to recognise that much still remains unknown about HRT given to populations different from those included in published studies. Trials produce generalised statistics of the risks and benefits of a particular treatment given to a particular population, whereas a woman seeking help for severe menopausal symptoms wants to know how HRT is going to affect her. We still need information from well-designed studies assessing younger peri-menopausal women taking HRT, particularly those with symptoms or those who are at high risk of osteoporosis. Furthermore, we need information about the risks and benefits of different types and doses of HRT: natural human oestrogens are not the same as conjugated equine oestrogens; non-oral routes may have different effects from tablets; and lower doses of oestrogen may have the same benefits as higher doses but with less risk.

Future research will help further to define the role of HRT and will also herald safe and effective alternatives to HRT. In the meantime, if you are taking or considering taking HRT, it is sensible to take the lowest effective dose of hormones and reassess your continuing need at least annually.

Questions & answers

• My doctor showed me how to examine my breasts for lumps but they feel lumpy all over. How can I tell if a lump is cancer?

Examining your own breasts is the best way to identify any unusual lumps or other changes. It is not unusual for breasts to feel generally lumpy without there being anything wrong. Ask you doctor or nurse to check your breasts first, and then feel them yourself so that you get to know what is normal for you. Then you will notice changes more easily.

Breast tissue is naturally affected by different hormones so your breasts will feel much lumpier during the progestogen phase of seq-

uential combined HRT, just as they did before your period during a natural menstrual cycle. The best time to check your breasts is just after a period has finished. If you are taking continuous combined HRT, you can check your breasts at any time.

If you find anything that worries you, check with your doctor. You should look for changes such as dimpling of the skin, changes in the nipple or any lumps that you can see or feel. In most cases, breast lumps are simple fluid-filled cysts and are not the result of cancer. However, if cancer is present, provided that it is treated early, it can often be cured.

• Since the menopause, I feel tired most of the time, have lost interest in sex and feel generally low. Can HRT help?

Symptoms of depression are common in the years around the menopause, so it is not surprising that hormones are blamed. Hot flushes and night sweats can disrupt your sleep leading to loss of energy and low mood. By treating the flushes and sweats, HRT can certainly help you to get the best out of life again.

However, depressive symptoms can result from many other significant events that occur at much the same time as the menopause – children leaving home, separation or divorce, and illness or death of parents. Depression resulting from events such as these will not respond to HRT.

If you have menopausal symptoms that are a problem, it is certainly worth trying HRT. If your flushes and sweats improve but you are still feeling low, it is unlikely that hormones are the cause and you need to look for other reasons. Some women may need both HRT and antidepressants at this time.

• My doctor has just started me on HRT. I was expecting to have blood tests or something to check my hormone levels but I was just asked lots of questions, given a prescription and told to make an appointment for three months' time. Don't I need any tests?

Hormone levels vary considerably and do not provide as much information as the symptoms you are experiencing. So your doctor is far more likely to ask questions than do tests! You will also be asked about your own and your family's medical history to ensure that it is safe for you to take HRT. If you are up to date with smear tests and mammograms, your doctor will not need to examine your breasts or do an internal examination, unless you have certain symptoms.

Once you have started HRT, you will usually be seen three months later to make sure that the type of HRT is right for you and to sort out any problem or concerns that you may have. When you are settled on HRT, you need only annual check-ups. However, if you have any concerns you should make an early appointment for review.

• Most of the studies recently reported have been about one particular type of HRT. Do the results apply to all types of HRT or just this one?

Many of the recent studies about the long-term risk of HRT relate to one type of oestrogen (conjugated equine oestrogen) and one type of progestogen (medroxyprogesterone acetate or MPA). In the UK, products containing these hormones are tablets called Premarin, Premique and Premique Cycle.

It is impossible to know if the long-term risks shown in these studies also apply to HRT using oestradiol and different progestogens. Clinical trials using different hormones and different routes of delivery are under way.

- My mother shrank as she got older and was told that her spine was collapsing because her bones had got thin. What can I do to prevent the same happening to me?

Your natural build, how much exercise you take and your diet will provide some indication of how likely you are to be affected. Thin women, who take little exercise and avoid dairy products, are particularly at risk, especially if they smoke. As oestrogen protects bone, the menopause, with decreasing levels of oestrogen, represents an additional risk factor.

Your doctor may send you for a bone density scan to assess your baseline bone density before considering treatment. If you are experiencing menopausal symptoms and are at risk of osteoporosis, you may be offered HRT. Otherwise, non-hormonal treatments available on prescription such as the bisphosphonates are the first choice to prevent osteoporosis in older women.

- I am 46 and my periods are very erratic but I'm not getting any other symptoms. Could this be the start of the menopause?

The first symptom of the 'change' or menopause is often a change in the pattern of periods, as you describe. Typically, periods will become more frequent and then they come further apart. You may skip one or two periods between otherwise regular cycles.

For some women, their periods cease with very few other symptoms. For others, flushes and sweats at first happen just in the week before a period and gradually become more frequent. Most women have had their last menstrual period by the time they are 54.

- I've heard all about a new type of HRT called Evista (raloxifene). What is it?

Raloxifene is not a natural hormone but is the first of a new class of synthetic compounds know as selective oestrogen receptor modulators (SERMs). These mimic the protective actions of oestrogen on bone without the unwanted effects on the lining of the uterus and breast tissue.

Clinical trials have shown that raloxifene can increase bone density, although not as well as conventional HRT. Raloxifene also seems to reduce the levels of cholesterol in the blood but there is no proof that this means that the risk of heart disease is reduced.

BMA

BMA Library

BMA House, Tavistock Square, London WC1H 9JP

British Medical Association
BMA House
Tavistock Square
London
WC1H 9JP

CERTIFICATE OF POSTAGE RECEIPT to be obtained and retained. You are liable for any lost items.

Raloxifene also appears to protect against breast cancer. However, much larger clinical trials are necessary to confirm this early finding.

On the negative side, raloxifene carries a similar risk of venous thrombosis (blood clots in the legs and lungs) as HRT. It does not affect menopausal symptoms and may even cause hot flushes. Overall, it has limited use in management of the menopause but may be useful for postmenopausal women at risk of osteoporosis who cannot take bisphosphonates or HRT.

- At 54 my periods stopped and I was lucky to have very few menopausal symptoms. But I'm now 57 and still experiencing severe hot flushes. I would like to try HRT but I have read that I would have to have periods again. Is this true?

Most of the commonly prescribed types of HRT for women going through the menopause combine daily oestrogen with a 10- to 12-day course of progestogen, which results in a monthly withdrawal bleed, similar to a period. But you can take both progestogen and oestrogen daily (continuous combined HRT) which should relieve your symptoms without a period. Tibolone is a single daily tablet that combines the properties of oestrogen and progestogen.

These methods are most suitable for women starting HRT several years after the menopause. They are not suitable for younger women because irregular bleeding is a common side effect. For milder symptoms, non-hormonal treatments such as phytoestrogens may suffice.

- Does HRT interfere with any other tablets that I take?

HRT is rarely affected by any other medication you might take. A few medicines interact with the way your liver breaks down hormones, which can make HRT less effective. This is more likely to happen if you take tablets for HRT than if you are using patches or implants. Medicines that might have this effect are some of those usually prescribed for epilepsy, such as phenytoin or carbamazepine. Some antibiotics have a similar effect. The herbal treatment St John's wort may also interact with HRT. Always check with your doctor if you have any doubts about what you are taking.

- I've read that HRT increases the risk of thrombosis. Do I have to stop HRT when I'm flying?

HRT increases the chances of having a blood clot in the legs (a deep vein thrombosis or DVT) or lungs (a pulmonary embolism). This means women on HRT are also at increased risk of having a blood clot on a long-haul plane flight, or in other situations where they are in prolonged cramped conditions. The standard advice about avoiding DVTs when flying is getting up and moving around regularly, drinking plenty of fluids and wearing support stockings during a flight. When seated in a plane, move your neck from side to side and up and down, and flex your ankles and wrists frequently – all to maintain good circulation.

- I'm 62 and I've taken HRT for the last 10 years. I'd like to stop HRT. Can I just stop it immediately?
Stopping HRT abruptly can result in a return of the symptoms. To prevent this, HRT should be tailed off gradually over two to three months under the supervision of your doctor.

- I'm 49 and started HRT six months ago. I was having terrible hot flushes before I started and my periods were all over the place. Although HRT has helped these symptoms, I'm not entirely happy with it. Whenever I take the progestogens each month I feel bloated and headachy – just like the terrible premenstrual symptoms I used to get with my periods. I'm not sure which is worse – stopping the HRT and getting the flushes back or continuing HRT and feeling so awful for two out of every four weeks. Is there a different type of HRT I could take?

Some women are very sensitive to the progestogen phase of sequential combined HRT, particularly if they experienced premenstrual symptoms in the past. Sometimes changing the type of progestogen, for example changing from norethisterone to dydrogesterone, can help. Otherwise, try changing to a sequential combined patch because non-oral routes contain lower doses of hormone compared with oral preparations. Progestogenic side effects are also less likely to occur with continuous combined HRT – partly because the dose of progestogen is lower when taken daily, and partly because continuous progestogen seems to cause fewer side effects than cycles of progestogen. Alternatively, consider the progestogen-containing intra-uterine system. Some women favour natural progesterone available on prescription as vaginal gels, pessaries or rectal suppositories, but drowsiness is a common problem.

Glossary

Amenorrhoea: the absence of menstrual bleeding.

Climacteric: the transition through the menopause.

COC: the combined oral contraceptive pill.

Continuous combined HRT: a regime of HRT involving daily oestrogen and daily progestogen. This 'period'-free regime is particularly suitable for women after the menopause.

Endometrium: the lining of the uterus, which thickens in response to oestrogen.

IUS: the intrauterine system, a device containing a rod of progestogen that is inserted into the uterus to provide contraception and reduce menstrual bleeding. It can also be used to provide the progestogen component of HRT.

HERS: the Heart and (O)Estrogen/Progestogen Replacement Study (HERS 1998). The HERS was designed to look at the effect of HRT on the rate of recurrent heart problems in women who already had heart disease.

HRT: hormone replacement therapy.

Licensed medication: when pharmaceutical companies develop new drugs, they undertake studies to assess safety and efficacy for the indication for which they developed the drug specifically. Once approved by the regulatory authorities, the drug can then be prescribed for this 'licensed' indication. However, once the drug has become widely used, it may be found to be safe and effective for a different condition. Doctors may prescribe the drug for this different condition, provided that the patient is aware that the regulatory authorities have not approved the drug for this different indication. Most doctors will prescribe drugs 'off licence' only if there is a specialist body that supports the use of the drug in that way. An example is the levonorgestrel intrauterine system (Mirena). In the UK, its licensed indication is for contraception and treatment of heavy periods. However, doctors have also found that it can safely and effectively be used as the progestogen component of HRT. Hence it is often prescribed 'off licence' for this indication.

Long-cycle HRT: a regime of HRT involving daily oestrogen and a course of progestogen every three months. This results in four withdrawal bleeds every year.

Menopause: the stage of a woman's life when she has her last menstrual period.

Mini-pill: a popular name for the progestogen-only contraceptive pill.

MPA: medroxyprogesterone acetate – a type of progestogen used in HRT and for contraception.

Oestrogen: a hormone produced by the ovaries. Deficiency of oestrogen after the menopause is responsible for most of the symptoms associated with the menopause.

Perimenopause: commonly used to mean the time between irregular periods and hot flushes starting and the years after the last menstrual period. Also called the menopause transition.

Phytoestrogen: plant-derived compounds with the properties of oestrogen. Typically found in soy and red clover.

Placebo: a treatment containing no active ingredients given to a person participating in a clinical trial in order to assess the performance of an active treatment.

Placebo effect: a measurable improvement in health in a person given placebo.

Postmenopause: the time following a woman's last menstrual period.

Premature menopause: the term given to a natural or surgical menopause before the age of 40. Women who have an untreated premature menopause are at greater risk of heart disease and osteoporosis compared with women whose menopause occurs within the normal timeframe.

Premenopause: the time from a woman's first to last menstrual period.

Progesterone: a hormone produced by the ovaries. Necessary to protect the thickening of the uterine lining (endometruim) in response to oestrogen, which if unchecked can lead to cancer.

Progestogen: a synthetic form of progesterone

Sequential combined: a regime of HRT involving daily oestrogen and a course of progestogen taken for two out of every four weeks. This results in 13 withdrawal bleeds a year.

SERM: selective oestrogen receptor modulator. SERMs are a relatively new group of drugs that include raloxifene (Evista). These synthetic drugs have oestrogen-like effects on bone, increasing bone mass and reducing the risk of spinal fractures.

SSRI: selective serotonin reuptake inhibitor. SSRIs are a group of drugs licensed for the treatment of depression and include fluoxetine (Prozac).

STEAR: selective tissue oestrogenic activity regulators. STEARs are a relatively new groups of drugs that includes tibolone (Livial). These synthetic drugs combine the properties of oestrogen, progesterone and testosterone.

Venous thrombosis: a blood clot in the veins, typically affecting the calves. Occasionally a blood clot from the veins can reach the lungs – a pulmonary embolus.

WHI: the Women's Health Initiative (WHI) study between 1993 and 1998: a set of clinical trials and an observational study set up by the National Institutes of Health in the USA. It was designed to test the risks and benefits of postmenopausal hormone therapy, diet modification, and calcium and vitamin D supplements on heart disease, breast and colorectal cancer, and bone fractures in postmenopausal women. More than 160,000 women aged 50–79 were enrolled as WHI participants.

Withdrawal bleed: when a course of progestogen is stopped, the resultant drop in hormone causes the lining of the uterus to break down and be shed as a withdrawal bleed or 'period'.

Useful addresses

Amarant Trust
41 Old Road
East Peckham
Kent TN12 5AP
Tel: 01622 870041
Fax: 01622 870041
Helpline: 0901 607 0312
Email: admin@amaranttrust.wanadoo.
co.uk
Website: www.amarantmenopausetrust.
org.uk

Provides information on hormone replacement therapy and runs a private clinic. Self-referral.

Benefits Enquiry Line
Helpline: 0800 882200
Minicom: 0800 243355
Website: www.dwp.gov.uk
N. Ireland: 0800 220674

Government agency giving information and advice on sickness and disability benefits for people with disabilities and their carers.

CancerBACUP (British Association of Cancer United Patients)
3 Bath Place
Rivington Street
London EC2A 3JR
Tel: 020 7696 9003
Fax: 020 7696 9002
Helpline: 0808 800 1234
Email: info@cancerbacup.org
Website: www.cancerbacup.org.uk

Offers an Information Service, staffed by specially trained nurses and supported by a panel of medical specialists, about all aspects of different cancers, treatments and related issues. Gives advice and emotional support to patients and families.

City of London Migraine Clinic
22 Charterhouse Square
London EC1M 6DX
Tel: 020 7251 3322
Fax: 020 7490 2183
Website: www.colmc.org.uk

Medical charity, working with St Bartholomew's Hospital, London for patients seeking specialist advice. Free treatment for NHS patients; a fee is charged otherwise. Doctor's referral letter required. As an unfunded charity, donations welcomed.

Family Planning Association
2–12 Pentonville Road
London N1 9FP
Tel: 020 7837 5432
Fax: 020 7837 3042
Helpline: 0845 310 1334
Email: library&information@fpa.org.uk
Website: www.fpa.org.uk

Offers telephone advice Mon–Fri 9am–6pm on contraception and sexual health. Appointment needed to view their reference library. Has a useful source of up-to-date information about other services and organisations relating to men's and women's health.

Institute for Complementary Medicine
PO Box 194
London SE16 7QZ
Tel: 020 7237 5165
Fax: 020 7237 5175
Email: info@i-c-m.org.uk
Website: www.i-c-m.org.uk

A registered charity formed as umbrella for complementary medicine groups. Offers information and British register of accredited practitioners, and recommends approved training courses. An SAE requested with two first class stamps.

King's Menopause Clinic
Menopause Clinic and Gynae-Endocrine Service
Suite 8, Golden Jubilee Wing
King's College Hospital
Denmark Hill
London SE5 9RS
Tel: 020 7346 8251
Email: hazel.mason@kingsch.nhs.uk

Menopause clinic in London open to women from outside the area. For information about the support group at this clinic, please write enclosing an SAE.

Relationship Counselling for London (previously London Marriage Guidance Council)
The Tavistock Centre
London NW3 5BA
Tel: 020 7580 1087
Email: info@counselling4london.com
Website: www.counselling4london.com

Runs counselling service for couples living or working in London.

Menopause Matters
Email: info@menopausematters.co.uk
Website: www.menopausematters.co.uk

Independent clinician-led website providing accurate information about the menopause and its treatment options.

National Institute for Clinical Excellence (NICE)
MidCity Place
71 High Holborn
London WC1V 6NA
Tel: 020 7067 5800
Fax: 020 7067 5801

Email: nice@nice.nhs.uk
Website: www.nice.org.uk

Provides guidance on treatments and care for people using the NHS in England and Wales. Patient information leaflets are available for each piece of guidance issued.

National Osteoporosis Society
Camerton
Bath
Somerset BA2 0PJ
Tel: 01761 471771
Fax: 01761 471104
Helpline: 0845 450 0230
Email: info@nos.org.uk
Website: www.nos.org.uk

Provides information, advice and support for people with osteoporosis. Helpline staffed by specially trained nurses. Has local support groups.

The Menopause Exchange
PO Box 205
Bushey
Herts WD23 1ZS
Tel: 020 8420 7245
Fax: 020 8954 2783
Email: norma@menopause-exchange.co.uk

Organisation offering publications and advice to its members. Details about membership supplied on request.

Relate National Marriage Guidance National Office
Herbert Gray College
Little Church Street
Rugby
Warwickshire CV21 3AP
Tel: 01788 573241
Fax: 01788 535007
Helpline: 0845 130 4010
Email: enquiries@relate.org.uk
Website: www.relate.org.uk

Do not have counsellors on hand, but can refer you to one of 100 branches. Have a bookshop and can provide a reading list on specific subjects. Relate publications available via mail order.

Women's Health
52 Featherstone Street
London EC1Y 8RT
Helpline: 0845 125 5254
Tel: 020 7251 6333
Fax: 020 7250 4152
Minicom: 020 7490 5489
Email: info@womenshealthlondon.org.uk
Website: www.womenshealthlondon.org.uk

Provides information on gynaecological and sexual health issues, through their helpline and leaflets.

Women's Health Concern
PO Box 2126
Marlow
Bucks. SL7 2RY
Tel: 01628 488065
Fax: 01628 474042
Helpline: 0845 123 2319
Email: counselling@womens-health-concern.org
Website: www.womens-health-concern.org

Offers information, advice and counselling to women with gynaecological and hormonal problems.

Publishes books and factsheets. Send an SAE for a current list of publications.

THE INTERNET AS A SOURCE OF FURTHER INFORMATION

After reading this book, you may feel that you would like further information on the subject. One source is the internet and there are a great many websites with useful information about medical disorders, related charities and support groups. Some websites, however, have unhelpful and inaccurate information. Many are sponsored by commercial organisations or raise revenue by advertising, but nevertheless aim to provide impartial and trustworthy health information. Others may be reputable but you should be aware that they may be biased in their recommendations. Remember that treatment advertised on international websites may not be available in the UK.

Unless you know the address of the specific website that you want to visit (for example, familydoctor. co.uk), you may find the following guidelines helpful when searching the internet.

There are several different sorts of websites that you can use to look for information, the main ones being search engines, directories and portals.

Search engines and directories

There are many search engines and directories that all use different algorithms (procedures for computation) to return different results when you do a search. Search engines use computer programs called spiders, which crawl the web on a daily basis to search individual pages within a site and then queue them ready for listing in their database.

Directories, however, consider a site as a whole and use the description and information that was provided with the site when it was submitted to the directory to decide whether a site matches the searcher's needs. For both there is little or no selection in terms of quality of information, although engines and directories do try to impose rules about decency and content. Popular search engines in the UK include:

google.co.uk
aol.co.uk
msn.co.uk
lycos.co.uk
hotbot.co.uk
overture.com
ask.co.uk
espotting.com
looksmart.co.uk
alltheweb.com
uk.altavista.com

The two biggest directories are:

yahoo.com
dmoz.org

Portals

Portals are doorways to the internet that provide links to useful sites, news and other services, and may also provide search engine services (such as msn.co.uk). Many portals charge for putting their clients' sites high up in your list of search results. The quality of the websites listed depends on the selection criteria used in compiling the portal, although portals focused on a specific group, such as medical information portals, may have more rigorous inclusion criteria than other searchable websites. Examples of medical portals can be found at:

nhsdirect.nhs.uk
patient.co.uk

Links to many British medical charities will be found at the Association of Medical Research Charities (www.amrc.org.uk) and Charity Choice (www.charitychoice. co.uk).

Search phrases

Be specific when entering a search phrase. Searching for information on 'cancer' could give astrological information as well as medical: 'lung cancer' would be a better choice. Either use the engine's advanced search feature and ask for the exact phrase, or put the phrase in quotes – 'lung cancer' – as this will link the words. Adding 'uk' to your search phrase will bring up mainly British websites, so a good search would be 'lung cancer' uk (don't include uk within the quotes).

Always remember that the internet is international and unregulated. Although it holds a wealth of invaluable information, individual websites may be biased, out of date or just plain wrong. Family Doctor Publications accepts no responsibility for the content of links published in their series.

Index